against all odds

CRAIG CHALLEN

AND

RICHARD HARRIS

WITH **ELLIS HENICAN**

against all odds

VIKING
an imprint of
PENGUIN BOOKS

VIKING

UK | USA | Canada | Ireland | Australia
India | New Zealand | South Africa | China

Viking is part of the Penguin Random House group of companies
whose addresses can be found at global.penguinrandomhouse.com.

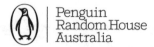
Penguin
Random House
Australia

First published by Viking, 2019

Cover photography by Heather Endall [top] and Lillian Suwanrumpha/Getty Images [bottom]
Cover design by Alex Ross © Penguin Random House Australia Pty Ltd
Typeset in Adobe Garamond by Midland Typesetters, Australia

Printed and bound in Australia by Griffin Press, part of Ovato, an accredited
ISO AS/NZS 14001 Environmental Management Systems printer

A catalogue record for this
book is available from the
NATIONAL LIBRARY OF AUSTRALIA
National Library of Australia

ISBN 978 1 76089 095 7

penguin.com.au

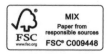
MIX
Paper from
responsible sources
FSC® C009448

To my mother, who taught me what is important in life. And to Heather, who has put up with a lot.

Craig Challen

For my father, Jim. He took a small boy out in a boat and ignited a passion for the underwater world that will last a lifetime.

Richard Harris

Contents

Foreword

The world was riveted by the news coming out of Thailand. Twelve local boys and their soccer coach trapped by early rains deep inside a cave system, cut off from the outside world, imprisoned in absolute darkness, with little hope of rescue. As rescue efforts escalated, ultimately bringing in thousands of rescue experts, divers, military and throngs of media, the situation only seemed bleaker by the day. The boys were found alive by two British cave divers who pushed through strong currents and zero visibility over four kilometres into the bowels of the mountain, but the rains were coming soon, which would wipe out all hope of extracting the stranded soccer team.

An outpouring of empathy from around the world kept the media spotlight focused on the mouth of that cave, where rescue workers, authorities, military, the distraught parents, and all manner of supporters and lookieloos had created an ad hoc city.

But a disturbing paralysis had set in. Yes, we know where they are. But how to get them out through miles of flooded tunnels?

As the hours ticked down, each plan seemed more desperate than the last.

Pump the water out? Rough mountain terrain prevented the kind of high-volume pumps necessary from being set up, and several people were injured trying. Dig a borehole down from above? Hundreds of holes were drilled, and none managed to sharp-shoot the cave the boys were in. Leave them inside until the monsoon season ended? But how to keep them warm, fed, healthy – and sane – for months, far underground? Teach them to dive and swim them out? But how could an assortment of average teenage boys all be taught the complex skills that cave divers took years to learn, in just hours, and in a remote, flooded cavern?

It was like a nightmare in slow motion. And it was in that nightmarish equipoise that Australian cave divers Richard 'Harry' Harris and Craig Challen joined the rescue effort.

The unique combination of their advanced cave-diving skills and their day jobs as doctors made them suddenly the most important members of the proposed rescue mission. That combination propelled them forward over just a few days from watching at a distance like the rest of the spellbound world, to becoming the tip of the spear of the final rescue. Why them? Because the more the rescue scenarios were analysed, the more it became clear that the boys would have to be somehow sedated, and brought out of the cave unconscious, for both their own protection against deadly panic, and for the protection of the rescue divers.

So the spotlight swivelled to the two guys in the international cave-diving community who were also experts in anaesthesia.

Now I'm not a cave diver. But I count a few top cave divers as friends, and I was taught cave diving by Wes Skiles, the famed *National Geographic* photographer, which is a bit like being taught to play tennis by Serena Williams. My couple of days diving the gin-clear spring-fed caves in Florida gave me more than enough respect for the divers who venture miles into flooded caverns – sometimes freezing, sometimes in zero-visibility water, and sometimes down to extreme depths – in their quest to see and explore beyond the limits of the known world.

I have enormous respect for the focus, intelligence, courage and physical strength required to do it. And as an explorer myself, I understand that illogical but irresistible urge to go as far from the warm, cosy centre of human experience as possible, to get to the very edge of what is known, and then go beyond it. If you've got that explorer gene, there is no thrill greater in life than to see that which has never been previously gazed upon by human eyes. That, first and foremost, drives us. A very close second is to survive and return to tell the tale. In my case, bringing back the images to support that narrative is also a very high priority, just below survival.

I've spent thousands of hours under water, many of them inside shipwrecks, at least 500 of them in diving helmets, another 500 in submersibles. I've spent more time on and (via my robotic cameras) 'inside' Titanic than the ship's captain did. And I've dived to the deepest spot in the world's oceans, seven miles down in the Challenger Deep.

But compared to some of the cave divers in this book, I feel like an amateur. They may differ in background and personality, but they all share the same rare combination of intelligence and grit. They survive the seeming impossible through an absolute focus on the task. They pit their wit and their stamina against the most fearsome physical environment imaginable. They understand the extreme risk they take diving under thousands of feet of rock, where the only way out is back the way you came in, and where there is zero possibility to simply swim to the surface if something goes wrong with you or your gear.

They manage that risk to its lowest possible value through intelligence, training and meticulous planning. But they can never manage the risk to zero. They accept the risk that remains, what I call the X-factor, because they are driven by the true explorer spirit.

Cave divers are some of the most self-reliant people on the planet. Even if you dive as a team, like Craig and Harry do, you're still alone on the dive. When squeezing through passages so narrow you can't wear your air cylinder on your back, with the rock pressing down on your spine and up on your belly, in water so murky you can't see your hand in front of your dive mask, miles in from the entrance, beyond all possible hope of rescue – you're on your own. The other guy might only be a few feet away, but he or she can't help you.

Cave diving is both highly technical and also the most primal human-mind-against-nature challenge that I can imagine.

I was initiated into cave diving by my good friend and co-leader of several of my deep ocean expeditions, Andrew Wight. Andrew was well known in the Australian cave-diving community, and possibly best known for leading an ill-fated expedition in the Nullarbor cave system in which the team became trapped inside by freak flooding and had to explore their way through to a previously unknown exit passage. He convinced me to make a fictional feature film, loosely adapting that story, which became *Sanctum*. In the process of producing that film, I learned a lot about the techniques, and the hazards, of cave diving. I also had to imagine, and bring to the screen, what it was like to be trapped by miles of solid rock, alone in the darkness with no hope of rescue. So I can extrapolate what it must have been like for those lost boys, in the days before they were found and as they waited to be rescued, and what it was like for the heroic divers who went in after them. Harry and 'Wighty' were friends, and hence Harry and I crossed paths on the set of *Sanctum* and in the *Deepsea Challenger* factory.

When I was reading Harry and Craig's story, I was biting my nails during some of the sections where they take us through the rescue dives moment by moment. Even though we all know that it ended well, it's important to remember that *they* didn't know that in the moment. Every decision they made was literally life or death, for those trapped kids, and possibly for themselves.

I was particularly struck by the soul-torturing ethical dilemmas each man faced as medical professionals. No one had ever drugged a child into unconsciousness, put diving gear on them, and then dragged them out through miles of flooded tunnels, including constrictions so small a single diver could barely slither through, blinded by silt, doing it all by feel. It's one thing to make decisions for yourself, as an explorer and adventurer, quite another to make them for a trusting and innocent child.

There was no precedent to what they were doing, and no guidelines for how it might even be accomplished. They were making it up as they went along, with the eyes of the world upon them. Not only the eyes of a fickle media, but also the eyes of the Thai authorities and the terrified parents. Imagine that dread weight upon their shoulders, as each decision was taken: what drugs to use? what dosages? and how to maintain that level of sedation? Additional injections would have to be administered throughout the multi-hour ordeal of the extraction. The rescue divers might even have to inject these kids through their wetsuits in some dark, flooded passage. They didn't know if they'd be bringing out corpses by the end of the dive. And if the first died, or the second, would you go on and inject that third kid and try it again? So many unknowns, so many variables.

It must have seemed like madness, but at the same time their relentless logic said it was the only answer.

In reading this book you'll live it, hour by hour, minute by minute, as it was experienced by two divers at the front lines of the rescue. Harry and Craig repeatedly stress how many skilled and heroic divers were involved in the rescue besides themselves – the British cavers who found the boys and helped with the extraction, the Thai Navy Seals who stayed with them in their subterranean prison and kept them healthy and hopeful, and many others.

Before it was finished, the rescue effort involved more than 10,000 people, including over 100 divers, 900 police officers and 2000 soldiers. A hundred government agencies from all over the world participated. But in the end it boiled down to a handful of skilled divers who swam those boys out. This book puts you there, deep inside that flooded cave, experiencing it first hand.

It is an inspirational story of what we humans are capable of when we come together to help others. It chronicles the international outpouring of empathy and effort to save those innocent lost boys. It is also an epic underwater adventure, the stuff of novels and movies, told in a humble, matter of fact way. But this isn't some Hollywood screenplay – this actually happened.

James Cameron, September 2019

Introduction

'They're All Going to Die'

Harry

It was the mission we'd all been training for, a life-or-death rescue in remote northern Thailand, deep inside a flooded mountain cave. The whole world was watching. The chances were disturbingly slim. Anyone who knew anything about cave rescue had to recognise that. Thirteen young people were huddled in the chilly darkness, one monsoonal downpour from the end of their lives.

And where was I?

I was 7022 kilometres away, at my usual post in the operating theatre of Flinders Private Hospital in Adelaide, making sure a thyroidectomy patient didn't wake up from her anaesthesia. I love being in theatre. But *man*! I'd never felt so far from the action in my life.

Early that morning before work, a message had popped up on my phone. It was from the legendary British cave diver Rick Stanton, who had raced to the scene to help save the stranded members of the Wild Boars soccer team.

'Could you sedate someone and dive them out?' he wanted to know.

Rick must be desperate, I thought. *Or the pressure of the rescue has sent him round the bend.* Otherwise, he'd never ask a question so absurd. Dive a sedated child underwater through the jagged maze of a dark, constricted cave? You'd kill the kid for sure. As an anaesthetist and a diver, the very idea sounded preposterous to me.

'Sedation not an option,' I replied.

It was Wednesday, 4 July 2018. Rick and I had been messaging back and forth for five days by then, ever since he and fellow British diver John Volanthen had arrived in Thailand to help guide the rescue. The boys had been trapped in Tham Luang cave since the evening of Saturday, 23 June – well over a week – and the outlook was grim. Rick hated what he found at the cave: a 'shit show' – Rick's phrase – of ill-trained adrenaline junkies, gung-ho military types, overwhelmed government officials and gullible, preening journalists from around the world sending out ridiculously optimistic updates about the chances of saving the boys. Things were such a mess on the ground, Rick confided, that he was ready to pack up his dive gear and fly home.

'Oh dear' was my two-word reply.

Thankfully, Rick and his guys decided to stay. They clipped on their tanks, spat in their face masks and pressed on. They would, of course, be the first divers to locate the twelve frightened soccer players and their 25-year-old assistant coach, shivering on top of a muddy hill more than two and a half kilometres in. But locating the team was one thing. Navigating the cave's narrow passages and sharp, jutting rocks in zero visibility to guide the boys out – that was something else entirely. That, I hoped, was where Craig Challen, my long-time dive buddy, and I might still fit in.

Ever since we'd seen the first stories about the boys lost in the cave, Craig and I had been angling to help. Both of us had trained for years in underground rescue. Both of us had decades of medical experience, too – I was an anaesthetist and critical-care doctor, and Craig was a veterinary surgeon. We'd played key roles in a couple of harrowing body-recovery operations. But so far, we had never been part of a live rescue involving so many people, or in such treacherous conditions as this, and no one had asked us to come to Thailand – *yet*.

So we waited at home in Australia, feeling anxious and irrelevant.

By this point, every man and his dog had a theory – not one of which was showing a jot of promise – about how to get these poor children out of the cave. Drill through the limestone from above. Pump the water out from below. Give the boys a crash course in scuba diving and swim them out. The billionaire tech promoter Elon Musk would soon be lighting up Twitter with his own creative schemes, which included an inflatable tunnel and a minisub. Or how about not bringing the boys out at all, but leaving them in the cave for the next five or six months, supplying them with food, clean water, space blankets and maybe some video games – and then walking them out after the rainy season? By the time Rick asked me about sedation, this wait-it-out idea actually seemed to be gaining some currency, a solid indication of just how perplexed everybody was. But if Rick was really serious about sedation as an option, I could think of a hundred ways it could end in tragedy and not a single way it might succeed.

'I should be over there helping,' I texted Rick, not for the first time. 'Craig and I are happy to provide any assistance.'

A couple of hours later, I heard from him again, this time making sure we understood exactly what we'd soon be signing up for. 'You're going to dive to the end of the cave,' he warned. 'You're going to see these kids. They're all looking healthy and happy and smiley. Then you're going to swim away and probably leave them all to die. Be mindful of that before you say yes with too much enthusiasm.'

Rick's words of warning didn't put us off. How could they? We knew we had to help. It was only after arriving in Thailand that Craig and I would fully comprehend what Rick was trying to caution us about. The plight of the boys was far more dire than any outsider realised. Only if exactly the right team of international rescuers could be assembled would these boys have a fighting chance, and even then they would need to rise to the challenge themselves if they were to survive.

Against All Odds is the true inside story of the greatest cave rescue ever, much of it revealed here for the very first time. The heartbreak and the triumph. The petty squabbles and immense satisfactions. The far-fetched strategies that were laughed out of Thailand and the one that would ultimately save the day. Most of all, it's the story of the remarkable band of characters who came together from around the world, hell-bent on saving these stranded boys no matter what the risk.

Rick and his mates, who looked like a ragtag collection of middle-aged hobbyists but were in fact world-class divers through and through.

Three Thai Navy SEALs who would turn out to be the greatest babysitters ever.

A charismatic Thai military doctor who would keep the children healthy, both mentally and physically, long enough to be saved.

The team's assistant coach, who would guide the boys through their ordeal with incredible devotion and a deep, spiritual calm.

Taken all together, it was quite a crew. And what about Craig and me? What could we bring to the scene that might save the lives of twelve young boys?

We weren't certain as we prepared to leave Australia, but we would soon find out.

I

Hoping

1

Making Harry

Harry

First, the name. Officially, it's Richard James Dunbar Harris, though pretty much everyone calls me Harry. Not Richie or Dick or RJD or anything else. Harry. My father was the only exception – for some reason he liked to call me Bert, but I never knew exactly why.

To end up in a remote corner of Thailand, helping to rescue stranded children from a flooded cave, first you need a strong thirst for life and a keen taste for adventure. I know exactly where mine came from – straight from my family, my dad especially. My parents were a classic doctor–nurse romance. My dad, James Dunbar Harris, did as many young Australian doctors did in the late 1950s and early 1960s, and travelled to England for specialty training, in his case from a talented vascular surgeon named Chris Savage. Once my father got to the hospital in Warwickshire, he met a doting ward nurse named Marion Taylor. They married in England and had my older sister Amanda there before moving back to Adelaide, where my sister Kristina was born. When I showed up in 1964, I was the baby in more ways than one.

From the time I was a little tacker, I loved being outdoors. My parents were happy to take my sisters and me on camping weekends and fishing in small boats. We knew people with beach houses. Every summer, we'd all get sunburnt on the sand. I loved swimming and snorkelling and trying to catch fish in the ocean. I wouldn't call those experiences adventurous exactly, just enough to plant a seed: the outdoor lifestyle was for me.

Dad was a huge influence. He was an affable, lovable, large-bellied bloke who grew up on South Australia's Murray River and enjoyed a glass of wine. His father and his father's brother had both died before the age of fifty from cardiac disease. 'I don't know if you should marry me,' my father supposedly said to my mother early on. 'I'll probably just die like my father and uncle did.' Given his family history, Dad chose a risky but understandable path. 'Well,' he'd say, 'if I'm only here for a short time, I might as well make it a good time!'

He had friends from every imaginable walk of life. Though he was a respected surgeon, funny characters were always dropping by. Tradesmen. Academics. Outdoorsmen. Some mate of his who was tinkering on a boat motor in our shed. Everyone had a story, my father taught me, and you should be open to all of them. He especially loved spending time with his birds. We had three backyard aviaries filled with parrots and other exotic species. I became his main bird wrangler. 'Bert,' he'd call to me, 'go in and grab that green eclectus parrot over there.' That's a big brute from New Guinea with one hell of a powerful beak.

'The eclectus?' I'd say, reluctant. 'They're a bit nippy, aren't they?'

'Just grab it, Bert,' my father would insist. 'We've got to give it a worming injection.'

I'd fetch the net and toss it over the bird. Then I'd hold it so my syringe-wielding father could inject the medicine into its belly, giving the bird every opportunity to chomp down on my thumb.

'*AAAAAAARGH! Dad, it's got me! Hurry up!*'

'Be gentle with it!' he'd snap.

'*Are you kidding? The thing just about took my thumb off!*'

Another typical afternoon at the Harrises'!

As I got a little older, I grew fascinated with snakes and lizards and other reptiles. 'Dad,' I suggested one day, 'why don't we dig up your rose garden? I could put my terrarium there.'

'No, Bert. We'll stick with the roses.'

He and my mother often had to yank me back from some crazy idea.

Mum was just as loving as Dad, but she could be a bit stroppy. She ruled the house. Maid Marion, we used to call her, or Winnie the Wettex, a tip of the hat to her beloved sponge cloth. She was constantly picking up after us and supplying us with food. If you wandered into the kitchen to help, she would shoo you out. Which left me domestically challenged and a little bit lazy, I suppose. My mother took care of everything.

I was an average student – bright, but cheeky and disruptive. I bristled under authority and liked to play around in class. I laughed whenever I got in trouble, which made everything exponentially worse. My best friend in school was Sam Hall, though he was far more studious and better behaved than I was. I was probably a bad influence on him. I became the extra son in the Hall family. I'd gobble up Mrs Hall's famous roast lamb and gravy, then go back home and announce: 'Oh, Mum, your gravy's not like Mrs Hall's.'

That didn't go over too well. 'Don't say that!' she'd bark, glaring at me.

Sam and I shared our first experience of true outdoor discomfort. There was a school camping trip that involved walking through the Adelaide Hills in winter with a backpack. We slept in a little tent. In the morning, we were given a map and compass and told, 'Off you go again.' We were absolutely miserable. It was raining and cold. No one could start a fire. There was no proper food to eat. The tent leaked, so the sleeping-bags got wet. I just about lost it.

'This is shit,' I moaned to Sam. 'I don't want to be here any more.'

But then we decided we'd just make fun of our miserable predicament. We had an expression we used over and over again: 'It's character-building.' When we got lost, it was character-building. When the sleeping-bags were drenched at night, that was character-building. Whatever bad things happened: character-building. We turned the whole thing into a joke, and that changed everything.

That was the first time I remember thinking, *How you react to something makes a difference*. It determines whether you're going to enjoy it or not. It determines whether you're going to be any good at it.

Pat Harbison was one of my father's friends. She was a renowned marine biologist. When I was about thirteen, I'd been out spearfishing in South Australia's Coffin Bay. I had speared half-a-dozen reef fish, which were very pretty to look at.

'Show me what you've got,' Pat said to me as I laid the fish out on the beach. 'What's this one called?' she asked.

'I don't really know,' I admitted.

'That's a zebra fish,' she said. She described what it ate and where it lived. 'You can't really eat it, of course,' she added.

'Okay,' I said.

She went through the fish one by one, teaching me about them and adding each time: 'Of course, you can't eat that one, either.'

Finally, a light-bulb moment. So I'd just murdered these six fascinating and beautiful fish for no reason at all. I was really embarrassed. Without any prodding or preaching, my father's friend had made me think, *In the future, why don't I just spear the ones we can eat?* From that day forward, I wanted to be a marine biologist.

I took an open-water diving course when I was fifteen and loved everything about it. Being underwater. Seeing the dramatic marine life – giant cuttlefish, blue-ringed octopus, red snapper. Learning about all the equipment. Also the fact that it seemed a little dangerous – that was exciting. On a warm, sunny February afternoon, Sam and I were in the Gulf St Vincent with Ron Allum, our diving instructor, and two young women. We were in fifteen metres of water, exploring the 1907 shipwreck of the *Norma*, five or six kilometres off the coast. We had a great time exploring the four-mast steel-hulled barque and were heading back to the dock around 5 p.m. when the waves in the gulf really began to kick up. We went down one wave into the back of the next, submerged and pitchpoled, flipping our small dive boat end over end and dumping all five of us into the water.

The boat was swamped, and the engine wouldn't start again. We were much too far out to swim back in. Fortunately, we were all wearing wetsuits and quickly donned life jackets. But all we could do was cling to the boat and wait. As darkness fell and the lights of Adelaide twinkled in the distance, the sea got rougher and the temperature started to drop.

This shows my naivety, but I figured the police boat would be arriving any minute to rescue us. Sam wasn't so sure. 'No one's coming out here tonight looking for us, mate,' he said. 'They'll wait until morning.'

'Don't be ridiculous,' I assured him. 'Of course they'll come. Mum and Dad are probably on the phone with the cops already.'

Sam and I felt like we were a little more resilient than the two young women. We cracked jokes and tried to get them to sing songs, but when one of them started praying out loud, we did feel a little unnerved. My mother, I learned later, had called the police, but they didn't exactly jump on the case. 'Oh, well,' the dispatcher sighed. 'You know young boys. They'll be off with some girls somewhere, probably.'

It was only at Mum's insistence that the dispatcher agreed to file a report. 'My son takes diving and boating very seriously,' she said. 'If he's not home when he said he would be home, there's a problem.'

Around 11 p.m., a police car swung by the boat ramp, where the car and the trailer were still parked. But the water was too rough by then to go out searching, even in the big police launch. We kept bouncing in the surf, holding onto the dive boat as the hours ticked slowly on. By two in the morning, no one was saying much of anything. We were half-frozen and uncharacteristically quiet. Around three, the floorboards of the boat began to pop out. Chunks of the buoyancy foam floated away. By then, even I was thinking, *This really might be it.*

At daybreak, we could tell we'd drifted with the tide. Down to the south, we could see boats and aeroplanes circling. Were they looking for us? We certainly hoped so. In the distance, we saw an old timber boat chugging towards us – *putt-putt-putt-putt-putt.* It was a beautiful sound. An old fisherman called out: 'Are you the blokes that are lost? Yeah, I thought you'd be about here.'

He'd looked at the tides and the winds, he said, and pinpointed us exactly. We climbed onto his boat, where he served us coffee and Vegemite sandwiches, then towed our waterlogged dive boat back to the ramp like a just-below-the-surface submarine.

I've always been proud of the fact that I went back to boating and diving after that harrowing night on the water. I decided the risk-reward ratio still tilted my way. Sam and I learned from the experience. We both became safer boaters, making sure we were always equipped with flares and a radio, and that the anchor rope was tied to the boat. I eventually did my coxswain's course and got my marine radio licence, but I still had a lot of growing up to do. I just felt lucky that my dad would still let me take his little boat and his camping gear and head out for another week of adventure, striking out on my own with my friends, getting away from our parents' supervision and testing ourselves.

One night when I was sixteen, I was behind the wheel of my mother's car, riding with three friends, when someone had a bright idea: 'Let's pretend to stage a kidnapping and give the crowd in front of the railway station a bit of a fright.' That would be hilarious, we all agreed.

So we dropped one guy off and then drove around the block. He was just standing there as we screeched up to the kerb. The others jumped out, pretended to bash our friend over the head and then tossed him into the boot of the car. Tyres squealing, we sped away. What great fun that was! In retrospect, maybe we should have anticipated the reaction we got.

An hour later, we were calmly cruising the city like young blokes do, arms out the windows, the radio up loud. Suddenly, we were surrounded by police cars. Sirens wailing. Plain-clothes cops jumping out. I can't remember everything, but I'm sure there were guns. 'Up against the wall,' one officer shouted.

As the cops grabbed and frisked us, I was still a bit confused, and I got a little lippy with one of them. 'What's going on, you guys?' I asked. It was only then that it finally occurred to me – this might have something to do with our lighthearted kidnapping prank.

The cops figured out quickly that we were just idiots, not dangerous psychopaths, but they still didn't find our joke all that funny. They'd already written up the media release with a description of the perpetrators and the car's numberplate. They'd already alarmed my parents, too.

'Has your car been stolen?' one of the detectives asked when my father answered the phone.

'My son's got it,' my father said. 'He's in town with some friends.'

My poor parents! I can still see their faces when the detectives finally hauled me home.

When it came time to apply to university in 1981, I was still keen to study marine biology. Then I spoke to one of my cousins, who was in his second year of marine biology up in Queensland. 'Don't do it,' he warned. 'There's no work. No one can get a job. The whole field is really depressed now.' So I went for veterinary science instead, choosing medicine as my backup. On school holidays, I had worked as a jackeroo on a sheep station near Broken Hill. I really liked animals. But I didn't get into the veterinary program at Murdoch University in Perth, the uni that Craig would attend a couple of years later. Instead, I ended up at the new and progressive School of Medicine at Flinders University, which had a strong commitment to public health around the world.

We had left-wing professors who wore skivvies to class. They'd practised in places like New Guinea or fought malaria in Africa.

And the campus was nothing like my posh private boys' school. Now I was studying with greenies and lefties, and some very ferocious young women who were more than happy to share their opinions on the environment, our male-dominated culture and women's rights. To them, I represented everything awful: a privileged white boy, the son of a doctor, who liked to drink beer in the tavern at lunchtime and head off on outdoor adventures in my breaks. I thought, *Oh, my God, I've never met anyone like these people before.* I was definitely out of my league. Arguing with them was like being hit over the head. Boys' brains at that age can be slow to develop, and mine was slower than most. For the first time ever, I could see what a sheltered, narrow upbringing I'd had. It was a bit of a wake-up call for me, a time to broaden my horizons. It took me a few years, but I'd get over myself eventually.

I made friends. I had fun. But that didn't leave much time for my studies. After I failed several subjects, I was close to being tossed out. I counted myself fortunate when I was called into the faculty office and told I would be allowed to repeat first year. I'm happy to say that, from that point forward, I never failed another exam. It hadn't come quickly, but I was starting to grow up.

I got to experience many different fields of medicine. Surgery. Paediatrics. Psychiatry. I liked anaesthesia. The art and the science of it. The fact that you really did hold the patient's life in your hands. But I also enjoyed travelling overseas and training in rural areas where there weren't too many other medical professionals around. In situations like those, I discovered, you were expected to do every-thing. Treat diseases. Perform surgery. Deal with public-health crises. Day after day, you really could save people's lives.

At Flinders, we were a small, close community, together for six – in my case seven – years, becoming doctors in our unique ways.

Despite or perhaps because of our extraordinary diversity – class, gender, culture, sexual preference, political outlook, nationality, ethnicity and just about any other category you could name – I really did become very fond of most of my classmates. And I never neglected my social life. I joined the university dive club, a well-equipped and active organisation. I became one of the dive instructors and was eventually elected president. One day in 1985, a few of us decided we were getting bored just swimming around the same old shipwrecks with the local fish, so we headed down to Mount Gambier in the southeastern corner of the state and signed up for a cave-diving course.

I can't pretend I loved it. It was wintertime, rainy and cold, and I was dressed in an old wetsuit. The water was around 15 degrees Celsius, and the cave was a grimy hole, full of weeds. The training was robust. We performed lost-line drills, how to cope if you lose your guide line in poor visibility. We learned exactly what to do when your regulator slips out. Half the time we were blindfolded. The course emphasised safety, which made sense, I suppose. But they had us in a very unpleasant environment. I couldn't help but wonder: *Why does anyone do this?*

There was a cave just down the road called Piccaninnie Ponds. Known for its crystal-clear water, fed by groundwater springs naturally filtered through limestone, the cave was famous for its striking green algae and pure white walls. The highlight of the course was going to be a dive in 'Pics'. Unfortunately, that cave was closed. The authorities were worried about divers disrupting the aquatic plants. So we never got to dive anywhere nice at all. When I got home, I joined the Cave Divers Association of Australia, mostly because I was eligible, but I never really got involved. I thought to myself: *I learned some things on the course, but cave diving is nothing I'll carry on with, that's for sure.*

A year or so later, I began spending a lot of time with a smart, pretty young med student named Fiona Allen. We'd known each other as friends and colleagues for two or three years before I started looking at her in a very different way. 'Cave diving?' she said to me. 'That's dangerous, isn't it?' I was still a very active diver, and I wasn't giving that up. But I was only doing bits and pieces of cave diving. I was happy to drop it entirely if she was worried about it.

Fiona and I married in 1990, and my life headed off in other directions, especially when our first son, James, arrived in 1996, followed the next year by Charlie, son number two. For a good, long time, cave diving just never came up again. I was getting my excitement in other ways. As a young doctor in training, I kept being drawn to what I would call the edgier side of medicine. At the Royal Adelaide Hospital and the Women's and Children's Hospital, I got to do some aeromedical work, flying off to emergency cases in a specially equipped helicopter. I finished my training as an anaesthetist at a small but busy district hospital in the northern New Zealand town of Whangarei. Part of that work involved flying into rugged environments without all the equipment and staff you'd find in a proper operating theatre. Cardiac cases far from any hospital. Vehicle accidents with multiple injuries. Serious traumas at far-flung worksites. Talk about life-or-death medicine! Those patients called on everything I had in me, providing a fierce rush of adrenaline. I always did my best, and I could usually make a difference.

'You're always dealing with people who are on the brink of death,' Fiona said to me one day. We worked in the same hospitals in those days. I was usually part of a resuscitation team, looking after peri-arrest patients. 'I'm happy to see you at those cases,' she said. 'You always look so calm.'

I didn't necessarily feel calm, but I realised then that I do have the ability to project a calm exterior even when everything around me is going to shit. If the person in charge is falling apart, a patient's chances can deteriorate rapidly. Someone has to at least *appear* in control. I don't enjoy those situations, but often I look back and say to myself: 'You know what? That turned out well.'

In 2000, I was working at the diving and hyperbaric unit at the Royal Adelaide Hospital. That was also the year our daughter, Millie, was born. Things were busy around the Harris house. One of the techs operating the hyperbaric chamber was a former police diver called Ron Jeffery. He said to me one day, 'Next time you go fishing down in the south-east —' which I was doing a bit of — 'why don't you pop into Mr Kilsby's property and have a dive in the sinkhole there? That's where the police divers do their training.'

I hadn't given much thought to cave diving in a while. But Ron sounded so enthusiastic, and he agreed to help set things up with the landowner. It happened Sam Hall and I had a fishing trip planned. Ron made the arrangements. I brought a scuba tank. Sam was happy to snorkel. He and I drove to the farm, found the sinkhole and jumped in. The water was freezing cold, but I had a wetsuit. I just went for a shallow, quick dive. And I was blown away.

The water was gin clear with a slight tinge of blue. The sun was shining down through the mouth of the cave. I went down about twenty metres, and the cave fell away below me. You can't imagine the clarity of this water until you've seen it. The Department of Defence used to use this sinkhole for testing the sonar buoys that are dropped from aircraft to find submarines. They had installed high-speed cameras in the sinkhole, at intervals, going all the way down, so they could drop a buoy from a gantry and then film it in slow motion as it plunged through the water. The water was so clear that they could see every detail perfectly as they watched the footage, never missing a thing. As soon as I climbed out of that sparkling water, I said to Sam, 'Oh, my God, what have I been missing? I didn't know it could be like this.'

I went right back and rejoined the Cave Divers Association. I managed to convince Fiona I wasn't going to kill myself and leave her a widow with three young children. I took the basic cave-diving course again. I was hooked. Soon, I was flying off to all the advanced courses I could find.

In 2004 Fiona and I left to spend two years living and working in Vanuatu, a former French colony in the Pacific Ocean that is now an independent island republic, part of an archipelago 1750 kilo-metres east of northern Australia. What Vanuatu lacked in modern sophistication, it more than made up for with beautiful, fascinating, water-filled caves. And I was, it seemed, almost the only person in the whole country who had any interest in diving them. I couldn't believe my good fortune. I had my own set of virgin caves. Most of them, no human being had ever set foot in. That's where I caught the real exploration bug. That was it for me. I was obsessed.

2

Making Craig

Craig

Like Harry, I had a circuitous route to Tham Luang cave. At an early age, I came to appreciate the thrills of outdoor adventure, but other things kept pulling me away.

My father, Bruce Challen, worked for a bank. Though he grew up in Perth, he spent the early part of his career bouncing from one country posting to another, living and working in each small town for a couple of years. My mother, born Patricia Patton, came off a farm in Trundle, New South Wales. While her two older brothers, Geoff and Harold, chose to remain on the land, their mother was especially keen on education for the girls, which was unusual for the time.

This didn't mean my mother and her sister, Pamela, had infinite possibilities. These girls weren't going to be lawyers or doctors or corporate high-flyers. Really, there were only two career options open to them.

Teaching or nursing? Which will it be?

These were smart, independent young women. *Nursing*, both of them announced. After finishing her training and working for a few years, my mother took an even bolder leap. She headed 4500 kilometres out to rugged Western Australia. And she didn't settle in relatively cosmopolitan Perth. She ended up in the north-western town of Port Hedland, where the only things going on were mining and cattle farming, and the women were few and far between. When this bright young nurse moved into town and showed up at the local hospital, everyone was very happy to see her – but no one more than the young, single manager at the local bank.

My parents married in 1963. I arrived, kicking and screaming, at King Edward Memorial Hospital in Subiaco in 1965, the first of my parents' four children – two boys and two girls. Three years later, Dad left the bank and took up a newspaper delivery business in the rapidly growing south-eastern suburbs of Perth. He did this for the next few years while we all went through our early years of school. But after all that time in the hinterlands, Dad felt constrained by the cushy sameness and convenience of suburban living. During my teens he bought a small farm in rural Gidgegannup, forty kilometres outside Perth, where we moved to raise sheep. It was a shock to the system, but we soon realised that the country was a fine place for kids to have adventures.

Despite my taste for the great outdoors, it was easy to feel isolated on the farm. My friends and I weren't old enough to drive yet, and there was no bus service, apart from the school bus. We had to depend on our parents for lifts. But that full-time move to the country turned out to be the formative experience of my life. It's where I really took to outdoor adventure. It's where I learned that whatever fun we had, we had to create for ourselves. The message was loud and clear: *Get out there! Just go do it!*

I would leave the house first thing in the morning with my brother, Ray, and not come home until dark, except maybe to check in for lunch. Our farm bordered a national park and the Avon River. So there were endless rocks to climb and paths to follow and other cool places to explore. We could head off in any direction – we'd find something there. And always there were jobs that needed doing on the farm. I don't know how else to put it: I just liked being outside.

Even today, I much prefer sitting on the open deck behind my house in Gnangara, a semirural suburb on the northern outskirts of Perth, gazing out at the property, instead of being cooped up in the air-conditioned living room. The smell of fresh air. The sound of the birds. All the plants and vegetation. It makes me feel alive.

I never had to work very hard in school. Good marks came easily, but I wasn't a sporty kid, something Harry and I share. I didn't show much talent for throwing, catching or kicking, and I was never really drawn to team sports. I much preferred hiking, riding and hunting for trouble with Ray and my mates. I just never cared enough to argue over which end of a paddock a ball belonged at. It seemed pointless to me. I knew long before I reached high school that footy and cricket wouldn't offer me a chance to shine.

From my father, I learned the importance of hard work and dogged determination. From Mum, it was the value of relentless inquiry, along with an openness to the opinions of others and a willingness to change. But my parents never pushed me towards any particular career. They just assumed that my brother, sisters and I would pursue something professional. My mother always made a point of saying, 'I want my children to make their own choices. You have to live your own life the way you see it.' And she actually meant it.

Like many young people, I had no clear career path in mind. I was perfectly content just being a kid. Luckily, as I began to map out my future, my everyday life was a guide. In the country and the suburbs, we'd always had lots of animals, and I was comfortable around them. We considered our dogs part of the family. I loved riding horses and had spent a lot of time working with sheep and cattle. I had an aptitude for science, and I enjoyed working with my hands. Being a veterinarian seemed like the obvious choice, though I almost blew my chance at it.

I hit a bit of a rough patch near the end of high school, just when it was time to decide what was coming next. I got distracted – that's what happened to me. I discovered cars and beer, at which point my studies seemed even less interesting than they had before. Also, the teenager in me didn't respond so well to authority. All I could think of was getting out of school and on with my life. I somehow knuckled down in the last few weeks of my final year, though, and did well enough in my exams to get into whatever university course I wanted. It was 1982. I was seventeen. I had to choose something. Animals, science, outdoors – so I went with the vet option.

I didn't have to travel far. A new public university had recently opened in Perth, incorporating a veterinary school. The first students had graduated only a few years earlier, in 1979. The School of Veterinary Science was Murdoch University's real crown jewel, a key part of what the new institution would become known for. Much of the southern side of the sprawling South Street campus was taken up by paddocks of livestock. The school had beautiful labs and research facilities. There was a full-fledged veterinary hospital right there, where students and academic clinical staff cared for all kinds of animals, from cats, dogs and birds to horses, cattle and even the occasional unlucky kangaroo. There were courses in wildlife, exotic pets and conservation medicine – and students helped to treat the lions, elephants and giraffes at the world-class Perth Zoo. Everything about the vet school sounded cool!

As it happened, my mother and father split up just about the time I was heading there. Their split wasn't especially bitter, and I didn't find it too upsetting. It might have been, I suppose, if they'd separated when I was younger. But Dad moved down to Perth, and I lived there with him for the first few years of uni until I could afford to move out on my own.

I had a great time in vet school. I could have studied harder – like many people at that age, I applied myself far less diligently than I should have – but I did well enough, and along the way I discovered that the part of the job that most appealed to me was surgery. I liked manual work, doing things with my hands, but I also discovered I had somewhat of a surgeon's personality. Surgeons are the swashbucklers of medicine. They get in there. They make a difference, and then they leave. The best surgeons are meticulous, intensely focused and sometimes downright obsessed, but they combine those qualities with a certain derring-do. It's a guts-and-glory pursuit. I didn't want to sit in a consulting room all day, performing check-ups, giving vaccinations and calming down nervous clients, whether animal or human. Surgery was where the action was, and where I wanted to be.

What vet school really taught me, though, was problem-solving and self-reliance. It is one of the best vocational courses for imparting those qualities. I gained skills there that would serve me well for the rest of my life. Much of the other stuff you will pick up on the job or not. Two months after graduation – *wham!* – you'll be standing in a paddock at three o'clock in the morning in the rain, trying to calve a cow.

I started my career as a locum, which was excellent training. I was often dropped in at the deep end and had to think and learn quickly. But soon I felt the stirrings of entrepreneurial instinct and was lured away from the profession to the world of commerce. I had a business importing and distributing foreign newspapers, back in the days when newspapers were thriving. I combined this with a newsagency in the city. Both businesses went well enough. I gained a great deal of experience in the business world, but I felt called to return to veterinary practice. In 1990 I took a position at Joondalup Veterinary Hospital. There, I was doing small-animal medicine with a smattering of horse work. That set me on the path that would occupy the next twenty-five years or so of my veterinary career.

By early 1993, I was romantically partnered with a young lady named Lianne Hulse. Between the two of us, we decided to strike out alone and start a veterinary practice. I did the clinical work, and she handled the management. At first, the practice treated a mix of large and small animals. But as time went on and Perth continued to grow, I was seeing fewer and fewer farm animals and horses and more family pets. It was a great area, and I derived a lot of satisfaction from looking after my wonderful clients and their pets. We had started the practice on a shoestring budget. There wasn't a cent to spare in the very early days. By day I did clinical work. By night I drilled, plastered, painted and whatever else was required in between after-hours calls from clients to get the place in reasonable shape. But with hard work it all started to come together. The practice thrived, and after a couple of years we started another a short distance away. A year later, we bought another one a little further north. Eventually we built up a network of clinics that would become Vetwest Animal Hospitals, the largest provider of veterinary services in Western Australia.

But though the business was doing well, by the time I reached my late thirties, I was starting to ask myself, *Hang on a minute here. Doesn't there have to be more to life than working? When does the fun begin?*

I didn't want to make the mistake my father had. There were many things to admire about Dad, especially his work ethic, which had stood me in good stead. But all he really seemed to do was work. I can remember only one proper holiday we took as a family. It was just a few days, and even then my father had to rush back to the business. My dad supported the family, which was important to all of us and, of course, to him, but he missed out on so many other things by working all the time.

As most people grow older, they become more and more like their parents. I vowed that wouldn't happen to me – or at least that I wouldn't miss out on fun, and other meaningful things in life, by working all the time the way Dad had. As the company grew and my role grew with it, I began to think about what really excited me. It wasn't being a veterinarian or a successful businessman, I realised. It was what I had first discovered as a child. It was challenging myself in the great outdoors.

Over the years, I had tried a range of adventures. Parachuting. Mountain climbing. Scuba diving. Motorcycling. Each of them had something to offer, its own unique, heart-pounding excitement. But I have to say: none of those captured my imagination in a truly life-changing way. All were fun, especially at first. But with each of them I ultimately concluded: *This is not a passion that will come to define me.*

The one that stuck was cave diving, which I first discovered in 1997.

Like Harry, I took a beginner's course. Unlike Harry, I took to cave diving immediately. I went on a few small dives to gain experience. My instructor and friend, Steve Sturgeon, obviously saw some sort of potential in me, because he invited me to join his cave-diving expedition to Vanuatu. I was thoroughly wet behind the ears, if you'll excuse the expression. I really had no business being part of that team. But I found myself exploring previously unknown caves. For the first time I experienced the thrill of seeing something that no human had ever seen before. I loved every second of the diving experience and vowed to do more.

Everything about it just appealed to me. Descending from the sunshine into the darkness. Not knowing what we would find. Checking the gear we had with us and checking it again. Squeezing through narrow passages and countless twists and turns. Paddling ourselves across the still, open pools. Discovering amazing geological formations. Trying to figure out where the water flow was coming from. Overcoming rapid currents, bracing temperatures, sometimes zero visibility. At other times, the water was amazingly clear. Managing what seemed to me like very complex diving equipment. Carefully unspooling the line that would guide us safely back home. Plus whatever nature threw our way. On that trip Steve had a serious accident during a dive and had to be evacuated by charter flight back to Australia, so I was also introduced to the dangers of this new activity. But I was unperturbed in my determination to pursue it.

An essential part of cave diving, I discovered, is amassing new gear. Soon, I was filling up a giant shed behind my house – a shed somewhat larger than the house – with tanks, regulators, wetsuits and drysuits, fins, compressors and other gas-mixing equipment, and every other kind of dive gear you can imagine. What can I say? It all comes in handy. And it's all to keep me safe. So it's easily justified.

The day I returned from one dive trip, I began planning another, if I hadn't started already. I was very fortunate during this period to be regularly diving with a couple of guys I'd met on that first cave-diving course, Karl Hall and Paul Hosie. Paul has gone on to become one of the most prominent Australian cave divers and explorers of the last twenty years. Both of these guys remain great friends of mine. The three of us learned deep diving in abandoned mines in the Goldfields region of Western Australia and made many visits to the Nullarbor Plain, an area famous for its beautiful and extensive limestone cave systems. The diving was spectacular and so was the camaraderie. Cave divers, as I would discover, are a predictably colourful and strong-willed lot.

I grew fascinated by Cocklebiddy Cave, one of the Nullarbor Plain's crown jewels and at one time the longest known cave dive in the world. I supported Karl Hall on his dive to the end of the cave in 2003. The cave is entered through a chamber over 300 metres long, leading down to a lake. This lake, about 180 metres across, is the entry point to a single, straight tunnel – 90 per cent of it underwater – that runs on for more than six kilometres. The first air-filled chamber in this tunnel is reached via a sump – an underwater passage – about a kilometre long. Once you've reached the First Rockpile Chamber, as it's known, you have to carry your dive gear across to a second sump, 2.5 kilometres long, leading to another air-filled chamber, Toad Hall. Then you carry your dive gear across Toad Hall to reach the third and final sump, which runs on for another 1.8 kilometres beneath the Nullarbor Plain. At this point you are 6.4 kilometres from the entrance. You then retrace your steps to return to the surface. Cave divers had been exploring Cocklebiddy for years, but I believe we were the first to dive it to the end in one continuous trip, which took a little over thirty hours.

By then, I was totally hooked. I *had to* explore these caves. How could I not? Our planet has some very tall mountains, some deep forests and remote deserts that are a million miles from anywhere – or might as well be. Yet at this point in human history somebody has been to almost all of them. But the unexplored caves? They are utterly virgin territory. Outside of space exploration, which is a little beyond my budget, what other outdoor activity promises that sort of adventure?

The only problem for me was finding the time.

As the years rolled along, my day job had become even more demanding. Vetwest was still expanding in the Perth area. We had also moved east and merged with an Adelaide-based company to form the Australian Animal Hospitals group. We had fifteen practices in Perth and four in Adelaide. I was very proud of all that we achieved. In 2015, the private equity firm Mercury Capital agreed to make a large investment in the company, which would allow us to double our size again.

Along the way, I had also grown close to the woman who would become my life partner, Heather Endall. Heather, a very attractive and highly accomplished person, is a force of nature in her own right. She had already had a long and successful career, initially as a veterinary nurse, then in sales and executive positions, before she joined Vetwest in an executive role in 2013.

The future was looking very bright. But by 2017, I had been running the company for twenty-four years, and I wanted more time for other things in my life, especially cave diving and aviation, my latest adventure activity. I had bought a helicopter and an aeroplane. I was enjoying flying both of them and learning about a new field of endeavour. So in January of that year, I left the office for the final time and retired as a veterinarian.

I thought about my father and reminded myself that very few people look back late in life and wished they'd spent more time in the office. I didn't think I would either. There were so many places I still had to fly to, so many caves just begging to be explored.

3

Teaming Up

Craig

It isn't true that all the serious cave divers in the world could meet inside a single school bus. It would probably take a small fleet of buses. But still, the global community of first-string cave divers isn't all that large. Most of us know each other. Or we know *of* each other. We know who the solid divers are – and who you'd rather not share a muddy sump with. Cave divers tend to be individualistic and self-reliant, the kind of people who like to push themselves hard and can tolerate physical risk. Inside a cave, you are responsible for your own safety and survival. But cave diving is still very much a team sport, a team sport for people who've always hated playing on teams. We're often together in remote locales for many days on end. We need help lugging equipment. We need people who can put up with the endless stories about our dive trips. We rely on each other's technical skill and support, starting with the crucial diver who lays the guide line that will steer us in and out of the cave.

Dedicated cave divers are constantly travelling the world in search of new holes to explore. But we do often dive with the same people over and over again. This is only natural, I suppose. When you're a hundred metres below the ground in a fast-moving current with zero visibility and nothing above your head but solid rock, your life really is in the hands of the friends you're diving with, especially the one who is your diving partner.

Harry and I had heard about each other before we'd ever met. This was 2005. We'd both been diving a while. He'd started before I had, but I'd stuck with it and he'd drifted away while he finished med school, got married and started having kids. We were introduced at a diving conference by Paul Hosie, the legendary diver from Western Australia who had been a fellow student with me on my first cave-diving course in the late 1990s and whom I had been hanging around with ever since. In 2006, Paul organised a trip to Kija Blue, a massive, azure-blue sinkhole in the remote Kimberley region of arid north-western Australia.

Kija Blue was stunning. Harry and I became fast friends.

I thought he was more experienced than he was. He'd really only come back to cave diving in the past few years. But with his large personality and professional skills, Harry was obviously capable. As our six-man team went deeper and deeper, the cave became tighter and siltier. At 111 metres, where a downward slope continued past a boulder pile, we knew we had a major cave system on our hands – and not enough time to dive it. We all left vowing to return.

I may have a higher risk tolerance than Harry does, but we both see the world in very similar ways. When we're trying to solve a problem, we may start with opposite points of view, but we respect each other's opinions as legitimate, and can always reach a conclusion together. These bonds are forged in the dark.

When it comes to our personalities, though, the two of us could hardly be any more different. Harry is louder and more talkative and loves making fun of himself. I am more stubborn, more focused and more single-mindedly intense. I'd say we're both pretty smart. I think I know what Harry would say about me. He'd say: 'My first impression of Craig was that he takes a bit of time to get to know. You have to earn his friendship. Craig doesn't suffer fools. If he thinks something is unjust, he will fight it as long and hard as he can.'

After returning to Kija Blue, we put together a trip to Cocklebiddy Cave on south-western Australia's vast Nullarbor Plain, where we managed to put 120 extra metres of line. We were in and out in a mad-dash twenty hours, eleven of them in the water. We didn't even sleep in the cave. 'A decent day at the office' was how I described that dive to one interviewer.

Harry and I shared an obsession with the Pearse Resurgence in New Zealand's Kahurangi National Park – deep, cold and dangerous. On one nine-hour dive, my 194-metre descent broke the depth record by 12 metres, a record previously held by Harry. He and I kept doing well together, and we kept coming back for more. Year after year, we leapfrogged each other's Pearse Resurgence dives: 207 metres, 221 metres, then finally 229 metres for Harry. We loved working out how to safely push our personal limits and the limits of physiology.

When Harry recounts our greatest cave-diving moments, he likes to feature, as he puts it, 'the many instances I've had to save Challen's life', often including 'that time on Christmas Island when we drove to the emergency department with him inside the boat, which was on the trailer still'. I would scornfully describe that same event as just one more example of Harry's meddling and excessive tendency to worry. What can I say? We have different recollections of certain shared experiences.

For Harry and me, cave diving has always been a hobby, sometimes an obsession, but never a job. We do it to challenge ourselves, and we do it for fun. The various records and other public notices are a by-product of going out in the bush and doing our thing, not the reason for doing it. Like life, cave diving is complicated and sometimes contradictory. Neither one of us wants to be mixing with a lot of knobs who are just blowing their own trumpets all the time. Diving together and with a small group of close friends has helped us both to avoid that.

Cave diving may or may not be the world's most dangerous sport. People debate this, and the answer really depends on how you measure it. Though the risks can be mitigated fairly easily, the hazards are obvious. Hundreds of divers have perished in flooded caves, including some of the field's most admired and highest-profile adventurers. Diving in a cave also tugs at some of the deepest human fears – drowning, darkness, isolation, being trapped. Cave diving is far more dangerous than open-water scuba diving, since so many more things can go wrong. In fact, it is about as different from regular scuba diving as scuba is from snorkelling.

Silt-outs. Floods. Rockfalls. Losing your line. Getting lost in the darkness and running out of air. Cave divers must be prepared for any and all eventualities and must never forget one life-or-death fact: panic and mistakes kill many more divers than geological surprises and equipment mishaps combined, which is why a big part of learning to cave-dive is learning to keep your cool, no matter what. And that can be tough. Panic thrives underground. It's dark down there. It's confusing. It's confined. It's hard to communicate. Rock is notoriously unforgiving. When you crash into it, it doesn't often move. Passageways can be stubbornly narrow and hard to navigate. The pressure keeps increasing with the depth. And in the overhead environment, a diver in trouble can't swim through rock straight to the surface for a breath of fresh air. The only way out is the way you came in.

Many of the world's most exciting caves don't look like much from the outside. But that out-of-the-way sinkhole or nondescript pond could easily extend kilometres underground, concealing an intricate array of underwater corridors and dramatic rock formations. And caves aren't just physically stunning. They are often powerful preservers of the past, time capsules that contain some of the deepest secrets of our planet and how it was formed.

The earliest cave divers didn't use any equipment at all. They climbed into the water, held their breath and swam as far as they could. Frenchman Norbert Casteret, a World War I veteran with an unquenchable thirst for adventure, made a bold free dive in 1923 in the Grotte de Montespan, where he discovered prehistoric drawings on a distant wall and secured his place as a hero to generations of cave divers to come. One of Norbert's trademark manoeuvres: tucking a candle in his oilskin cap to light his passage beyond the stygian darkness of the sump. No one could possibly discount the bravery – or lung capacity – of such fearless pioneers. But the human body, no matter how practised or how strong, is a severely limited instrument in the absence of air. Trying to breathe water has a 100 per cent failure rate, no matter who's sucking it in.

Today's cave diving owes its existence to the forward march of technology. Without some way to breathe beneath the surface, no cave diver could ever get very far. The dawn of the modern age can be traced to 4 October 1936. That morning, Jack Sheppard, a telecommunications engineer at the post office in Bristol, England, stepped into a homemade drysuit and hooked himself up to a bicycle pump with a flexible hose, a tobacco-tin stopper and a rubber mouth-piece, all held together with metal clips. It was a cartoonishly clumsy contraption. But this rudimentary breathing machine delivered sufficient oxygen to carry young Jack through sump 1 of Swildon's Hole, part of an extensive spring-fed cave system thirty-two kilo-metres from his home. Later that year, Sheppard's respirator became self-contained when he and his diving partner, Francis Graham Balcombe, connected the kit to an oxygen cylinder. At that point, their trips were no longer limited by the length of the rubber hose.

Word of these early adventures spread quickly. *Cave diving!* People were excited at the very idea. Some of those pioneering dives were broadcast live on BBC radio. That's how much interest there was.

World War II left a vast surplus of underwater-warfare equip-ment: oxygen diving cylinders, soda-lime absorbent canisters and, especially, body-hugging frogman suits. The suits were especially welcome in Britain, where the underground water temperatures tended to hover around 12 degrees Celsius. When legendary divers Jacques Cousteau and Émile Gagnan invented the aqualung in 1943, it seemed like it might be the ticket to deeper, flooded chambers. But three years later, Cousteau nearly died from carbon-monoxide poisoning while searching for the bottom of the spring at Fontaine-de-Vaucluse in south-eastern France. That same year, Sheppard and Balcombe formed the Cave Diving Group, to provide divers with better training. The CDG became a centre of cave-diving knowledge and remains active today.

Despite the patchy knowledge and ragtag equipment, these divers kept pushing ahead. By 1960, modern wetsuits offered a much-improved mix of buoyancy and insulation. Side-mounted cylinders made it easier to move underwater, as cave divers squeezed their bodies through narrower and narrower openings. Visibility was improved, too, with more intense helmet-mounted lights. As the divers grew more confident swimming underwater, they extended their range even further by donning fins.

By the mid-1960s, organised cave diving was beginning to spread around the world, especially to Australia, New Zealand and the US, thanks to the passions of two classes of adventurers: open-water scuba divers who wanted to test their skills in a more complex underground environment, and cavers who didn't like calling a halt to their explorations at the water's edge. But training was sorely lacking. After an early rash of deaths in the 1970s, American Sheck Exley, the first chairman of the Cave Diving Section of the National Speleological Society, published *Basic Cave Diving: A Blueprint for Survival*, which helped establish some useful procedures and calmed everyone down. Ironically, Exley was killed in 1994 at age forty-five trying to set a depth record in the world's deepest sinkhole, Mexico's 330-metre Zacatón. His wrist-mounted dive computer indicated that he'd reached a maximum depth of 276 metres.

The rise of professional instruction pushed safety as priority number one, and cave-diving equipment was finally being standard-ised. Advances and refinements in equipment configuration helped to 'keep it simple and streamlined'. Following the 'rule of thirds' became the norm: you use no more than a third of your air on the way into the cave, leaving a third for the trip out and the final third as a safety reserve. Carrying more than one cylinder, each with an inde-pendent demand valve, also became standard practice, meaning that a diver in trouble would always have a backup. These basics would save countless lives over the years. Violating them would prove fatal time and time again.

*

Such was the state of cave diving when Harry and I showed up in the 1990s. Divers had made great advances. So had the gear. But the possibilities were about to explode again with the arrival of the so-called technical diving revolution. Truly, the fun had only just begun.

Here's how I like to explain it: everyone knows about regular scuba diving, the kind you do in the ocean when you're on holiday, swimming around, looking at fish and coral. The water is relatively shallow. There's often a reef nearby. You carry a single tank on your back, filled with air from a compressor supplied by the local dive shop. You breathe in through a regulator. You breathe out into the water, sending a rush of bubbles up to the surface. Once the tank's getting low, you follow the bubbles and call it a day. Then it's beer o'clock.

Technical diving is different. It often means diving in an area where your free ascent to the surface is somehow blocked. Maybe you're inside a shipwreck. Maybe it's a mine or a cave. Maybe there's an artificial ceiling imposed by the need to stop and decompress, eliminating gases accumulated in the body under pressure in order to prevent decompression sickness or 'the bends'. Whatever it is, you can't swim straight up when you are done. Getting safely out of there requires special techniques and gear. By the time Harry and I started diving, people had begun experimenting with different mixes of oxygen, nitrogen and helium to extend the dives and make them safer. Rebreathers are manually or electronically controlled devices that allow you to breathe the same air repeatedly by adding oxygen and removing carbon dioxide from your inhaled air, allowing you to dive deeper and stay longer. The masks and the fins hadn't changed much. But the exposure suits, as we call them, were always improving. Wetsuits, drysuits, new concepts and new materials. There is a suit – often many suits – for almost any dive. Like most divers, Harry and I have a whole collection of exposure suits hanging at home. Several wetsuits, a couple of drysuits. Thin ones, thick ones and some in between.

But why would anyone want to dive in a cave?

We've been getting that question for years. I used to say: 'If you need to ask the question, you wouldn't understand the answer.' For me, it's never been entirely logical. It's more a compulsion or an urge. It's no different, I suppose, from trying to explain to someone the merits of skydiving or mountain climbing or bouncing around in a whitewater raft. If it doesn't call to you, I probably can't convince you to love it.

Curiosity is surely part of the equation. Cave divers are the kind of people who can't leave well enough alone. If I'm walking through the bush and I see a hole in the ground, I really need to know: 'How deep is that hole? How far does it go? Does it go straight down or veer to the side? Where does the water in it come from?' I'm not sure why questions like those tug at me, but they do. For Harry, it's about exploration, but it's also about bringing back video and images to share with others.

Challenge is another part of cave diving's appeal. If anyone could do it, it wouldn't be nearly so much fun. There wouldn't be the feeling of accomplishment, the satisfaction of doing something hard. Cave diving can be logistically complicated, physically gruelling and potentially dangerous – all the things that cavers love.

Technical fascination is part of it too. Divers tend to be technically minded people. We have to have the latest gear. We are constantly testing new equipment – how to prepare it, how to repair it and how to improve on it. That's a key part of the fun. But the biggest attraction in cave diving, I believe – the thing that keeps most cavers coming back for more – is the inherent excitement of exploration, the unyielding desire to go somewhere no one has gone before, the thrill of possibly discovering something new.

There are precious few opportunities in this life to go somewhere that no human being has ever gone before or to see something that has never previously been seen. To me, that's just such a privilege. When you've had the chance to do it, you want to do it again.

Of all the dives Harry and I have taken together, the one that prepared us best for Thailand was our saddest dive of all.

Agnes Milowka was a rising star of cave diving and a great friend of ours, an extremely talented and self-assured young Australian diver. Born in Poland, Agnes had moved to Melbourne as a child and studied maritime archaeology at Flinders University. She had done a lot of wreck diving, then discovered the thrill of cave diving and shot right up the ranks. 'I dream about caves,' she said early on.

Still in her twenties, she made amazing discoveries in the caves of Mount Gambier. She earned an internship in Florida and began making discoveries there, laying much fresh line. She caused some controversy because she would sneak into the caves by herself after work. More than once, people saw her car parked outside and grew alarmed: 'Oh, someone hasn't come out of the cave.' But that was Agnes, pushing fast and hard. On an expedition to Cocklebiddy Cave in Western Australia, she reached the midpoint of the line I had laid in 2008, giving her the record for the longest cave dive in Australia for a female.

'Take it easy,' several of us urged her. 'There's plenty of time. Don't rush things. Just be careful.' But she was young and didn't give much thought to her own mortality. There were so many amazing caves she still had to explore.

Agnes wrote articles, gave speeches and worked with *National Geographic* and the Discovery Channel. She was a stunt diver on James Cameron's 3D diving film, *Sanctum*, which she described on her website as the story of what can happen when a dive 'goes terribly wrong'. 'Inside a cave system,' she wrote, 'the line between life and death is a fine one, which naturally makes for thrilling adventure.'

Agnes made a few comments that, frankly, worried Harry and me. 'You'd have to be stupid to die in Mount Gambier in those simple caves,' she told us one day, which was maybe a little insensitive to the twelve or thirteen people who had died there over the years.

But we loved Agnes. Everybody did.

Fast-forward to February 2011. The caves of Piccaninnie Ponds, twenty kilometres west of Mount Gambier. When Harry came up to the surface, he was told that someone in the group was overdue coming out of nearby Tank Cave. Tank Cave is only around fifteen metres deep, but it's a complex maze with eight kilometres of interwoven tunnels and tight restrictions. He had the sinking feeling: *It's going to be Agnes.* She had asked some of the guys about good places to prospect for new leads, and they'd told her about a spot they'd been scratching away at for years, very slowly moving a few rocks at a time so they could get a little further in, proceeding carefully, like they were trained to.

As well as we could piece together later, Agnes had bowled into a hole leading to a new passage about 600 metres from the entrance and kept going, squeezing through some extremely narrow openings. She was small, and famous for pushing through tight, restricted country. At one point she had taken off one of her cylinders to push herself further in. That's a risky manoeuvre. You've dropped your redundant gas supply. If anything goes wrong with your other tank, you're in serious trouble.

Going further into the cave, she'd turned around and got lost in the silt. She never made it out.

It was a group effort to find Agnes's body. One team of divers followed the line she had laid, then Harry and another diver pushed through some very tight country until they came upon her discarded cylinder. Not far away, Harry spotted Agnes's body. It was perpendicular to the line, suggesting she'd been trying to go out through a tiny crack that didn't lead anywhere. It looked like Agnes had still been fighting right to the end. Her gear was all undone. She was obviously trying to take stuff off and fit through this little hole, in zero visibility as she had stirred up a lot of silt during her entry, which you would expect in these tight conditions. When the gas ran out, she had returned to within three metres of her other tank, but she was pointing in the wrong direction.

I arrived from Perth the next day after Harry called me in to help. For three days, working in buddy pairs, we and other divers dug out the cave to reach her body and retrieve her gear. Harry did the last dive, pulling Agnes's body out to a spot where I was waiting, about five metres back. From there Harry led us out. I followed, pulling Agnes behind me.

As we moved along this tiny, flat tunnel, Harry floated up off the floor a little and ended up in a sort of blind alcove in the roof of the cave. Neither of us could see anything, and I had no idea what was happening. I kept moving forwards, pushing Agnes ahead of me, squashing Harry from behind, trapping him, as he tried to work out why the tunnel had just stopped. He had to push Ag back at me, so I'd reverse out and we could continue on. A very simple error could have been a major problem. Harry told me later he really had to fend off some rising panic there. That's a risk and often a reality in any rescue or recovery.

Agnes's loss was a tragedy for us, but her memory lives on. That May, she posthumously received the Exploration Award from the National Speleological Society Cave Diving Section in recognition of her outstanding and dedicated service. At least three geological features have been named in her memory: Ag's Dreamtime Tunnel in Olwolgin Cave on the Nullarbor Plain, and in Victoria, Agnes Chamber in the Davies Cave System at Bats Ridge, and Milowka Canal in Elk River Cave.

'There is no greater feeling in the world than finding a passage that no one ever in the history of the world has seen before,' Agnes said in one of her many YouTube videos. 'It is like any pursuit that is inherently dangerous. If you are pushing the boundaries of that sport, you will find yourself taking on bigger and bigger risks. To me those risks are worth it, because the rewards are worth it.'

I just wish she were still around to enjoy more of them. She was only twenty-nine years old.

4

Lost Boys

Craig

Good news travels slowly, even in this digital age of ours. But crises and catastrophes? They zoom across the oceans at lightning speed. Especially when the story involves a group of young people as endearing and photogenic as the stranded members of Thailand's Wild Boars soccer team. It was impossible to hear their heart-wrenching story or see pictures of such fresh-faced boys and not feel an instant, human connection to them.

Were these children really going to die?

No wonder the international media highlighted their plight with round-the-clock updates. No wonder millions – *billions?* – of TV viewers hung on every detail, hoping against hope that the boys would somehow make it out alive. In a cynical, deeply divided world where hardly anyone can agree on anything, here was a news story where there could only be one side. It's not too much to say that for a couple of nerve-racking weeks in the middle of 2018, a badly fractured planet was briefly united by the life-or-death drama playing out in a remote cave in Thailand.

When the story first hit the news, Harry and I were at home in Australia, going about our daily lives. Harry was looking after his patients in Adelaide and trying to keep up with Fiona and their three nonstop kids. I was enjoying my early retirement in Perth, hanging around with Heather, flying my plane and my helicopter and trying to keep fit by clocking up miles on my bike. Harry and I were about to leave on a ten-day cave-diving trip to the Nullarbor Plain. If we were glued to the reports from Thailand more closely than most people, that was for two reasons, I suppose. Though we had never dived in Tham Luang cave near the Thai border with Myanmar, we'd been inside caves like it, and we knew many of the divers engaged in the search or who would soon be flying in to participate in the rescue. Oh, and one other thing: we had enough cave-diving knowledge and experience to realise just how daunting this mission would be. Most cave-diving rescues end as body recoveries. That's just a fact. As we exchanged emails, texts and phone calls with each other and with other divers around the world, almost everyone seemed to agree: these precious young people were highly unlikely to come out of that cave alive.

The trouble all started, as trouble often does, in the most mundane way imaginable. It was a humid, cloudy Saturday in the far-northern Mae Sai district of Thailand's Chiang Rai province. The boys of the Moo Pa ('Wild Boars') youth soccer program had just finished their weekend practice and split up into two squads for a club friendly. After coming off the field, a dozen of the young players, ages eleven to sixteen, decided to make one last stop before heading home. One of the boys, Pheeraphat Sompiengjai, known by his nickname 'Night', was celebrating his sixteenth birthday that day, making him the oldest player on the team. Night's parents had a bright-yellow SpongeBob SquarePants cake waiting for him at home. But the boys wanted to hold their own small celebration.

They rode their bikes from the practice field through rice paddies and forested hills to Tham Luang cave, about twenty minutes away from the field. Their young assistant coach, Ekkapol Chantawong ('Coach Ekk'), agreed to come along. The boys stopped on the way for some snacks and juices. Outside the cave, they carefully lined up their bikes against a rail, dropped their backpacks in the dirt and traded their soccer shoes for thongs and sneakers. Together, they hiked excitedly inside.

'Just a short visit,' Coach Ekk cautioned. 'Then, everyone must go home.'

Later, people around the world would second-guess that decision, describing it as reckless or worse. Some commentators would ask how a 25-year-old assistant coach could possibly allow these children to make such a risky journey. But when you grow up in the foot-hills along the Thai–Myanmar border, visiting the cave isn't that big a deal. The cave is a local tourist attraction. Most of the players had been there before. They'd even conducted initiation rituals inside one of the deeper chambers, writing the names of new team members on a flat limestone wall. Until the monsoon season arrived each summer, a short visit to the cave wouldn't spark any alarm at all. Some more cautious than the dozen young, athletic soccer players might have hesitated outside the mouth of the cave, where a sign warned in English and Thai: 'DANGER! FROM JULY – NOVEMBER THE CAVE IS FLOODING SEASON.' Then again, July was still eight days away. Though it had been raining on and off for the past three days, there was no sign of flooding at the mouth of the cave when the coach and the boys, most of them still dressed in their soccer jerseys and shorts, with a few cheap headlights to illuminate the way, advanced through the first chamber and hiked deeper inside.

In the rich folklore of northern Thailand, there are many stories about these cloud-swathed mountains and the caves that snake beneath them – the Tham Luang–Khun Nam Nang Non, as this underground system is officially called. That means 'the Great Cave and Water Source of the Sleeping Lady Mountain'.

It is said that in ancient times a beautiful princess fell in love with a stableboy and became pregnant by him. Knowing their love was forbidden, the young couple fled their families and went into the cave to hide. When the stableboy left in search of food, he was caught by the army of the princess's father and killed. When her beloved failed to return, the princess stabbed herself and bled to death in the cave. As legend has it, the surrounding mountains took the shape of the princess's body. Her blood became the water that flows through the cave. To this day, her spirit is said to inhabit the cave's many underground chambers and passageways, holding powerful sway over all who enter.

It took a couple of hours for the boys' parents to grow concerned. By then, the rain had begun to fall again. This time, it was hard and steady and didn't let up. Around 7 p.m., as darkness was falling, Wild Boars head coach Nopparat Khanthawong checked his phone and found more than twenty missed calls and voice messages, all of them from parents worried that their sons had not come home. Nopparat dialled his assistant, Coach Ekk, as well as several of the missing boys. No one answered. Eventually, though, the head coach reached one of his other players, thirteen-year-old Songpol Kanthawong.

'Do you know where Ekk is?' the coach asked frantically. 'Do you know where the boys are?'

'They went to the cave,' Songpol answered. He had planned to go along, he said, but he'd got a last-minute call from his mother, who insisted he return home with the motor scooter he had ridden to soccer practice that day. She needed the scooter for work. Reluctantly, Songpol had told his friends goodbye.

The head coach drove straight to the cave, where he spotted his players' bikes and backpacks strewn on what was now a muddy path. He quickly concluded the obvious: Ekk and the boys had gone into the cave and not come out. The coach called the authorities immediately and then alerted the worried parents, who started arriving soon after the police and paramedics did, joined by some Thai soldiers, and then park rangers from the public authority that oversees the cave. But with the rain still coming down and the water pouring in, no one had a clear idea of what to do if the Wild Boars were lost somewhere in the twisted depths of Tham Luang cave. Where exactly were they? And more to the point, how could the eager first responders possibly get to them in the labyrinthine cave?

The park rangers made tentative forays inside, but they didn't get too far. Though the first part of the cave was dry, they quickly came upon a T-junction where the water had risen too high for them to pass. Carrying on seemed impossible, at least until the rain subsided and the water flow slowed a bit. All anyone could hope was that the boys hadn't been washed away in the rising floodwaters – that they'd found a dry ledge or some other pocket of safety to wait out these dicey hours.

By the next morning, the crowd outside the cave had begun to swell with a fresh wave of Thai national police officers, military personnel and concerned local residents, all eager to be helpful. They joined the first responders and anxious relatives who had stayed all night, waiting for snatches of information that never arrived. Among the newcomers was Vern Unsworth, a British caver based in Chiang Rai, an hour's drive south of the cave.

News crews gathered as well, their satellite trucks and other equipment parked along the road that led to the cave. Many more of them would soon be coming as the story of the lost boys spread. Slowly, details about the boys' lives began creeping into the media, along with photos from their Facebook pages and from classmates' mobile phones. Mark was the smallest, though not the youngest. Titan, the youngest, was deathly afraid of the dark. Dom's mother ran a clothing stand in the Mae Sai market. Five of the boys attended Mae Sai Prasitsart School. Ever so gradually, the Wild Boars were coming to life in the public's mind, moving from a generic group of Thai children – 'the boys' – to individuals with distinct personalities and special family circumstances. Coach Ekk and three of the boys, Adul, Mark and Tee, the media reported, were not actually Thai citizens. Though born in Thailand, they came from ethnic groups who for generations have moved across borders in the remote hills of China, Myanmar, Laos and Thailand. Like half a million others in Thailand, these so-called stateless people are denied many of the basic rights of citizenship.

Ekk's story was especially tragic. In 2003, when he was just ten years old, an epidemic swept through his tiny village, killing his mother, father and seven-year-old brother and sparing only him. A sad and lonely boy, Ekk was taken in by relatives, who sent him to a Buddhist temple, where he trained to be a monk. He shaved his head, wore saffron robes, learned to meditate and studied the Tripitaka, the Mahayana sutras and the Tibetan Book of the Dead, the three major Buddhist texts.

Ekk was said to have moved out of the temple about five years ago, to care for his ageing grandmother, and that's when he became the Wild Boars' assistant coach. He loved the boys, everyone agreed, and gave generously of his time and attention, often looking after them when their parents were busy or away.

Some in the media questioned why a young adult would lead a dozen children into a cave, allowing them to get stranded in a flood. But none of the parents seemed to blame the coach at all. 'I would be so much more worried if Coach Ekk wasn't with them,' one of the fathers said. 'He will do whatever he must to keep them safe.'

Outside the cave, the mood was growing increasingly tense as fear for the boys' safety mounted. 'My son, come out,' cried Titan's mother. 'I am waiting for you here.'

'Please hurry and come home,' wailed another, whose son, Biw, was the team's goalie. 'My son, let's come home together.'

The mother of a boy named Dom began to weep as soon as she recognised her son's bike and soccer bag. 'My heart is gone!' she cried.

One of the fathers was obviously torn. 'I am not sure if we will find them today if it keeps raining,' he said. 'But I asked for all God's wishes. I am certain that they will survive.'

The father wasn't alone in seeking intercession from above. In this region, beliefs are heavily influenced by Buddhist, Brahmin and animist traditions. Several red-eyed parents gathered in a sombre prayer ceremony led by an elderly saffron-robed monk, accompanied by the slow, haunting beat of a small drum. Classmates of the boys held a group prayer session of their own, singing songs of encouragement, folding paper cranes and posting hopeful messages on their Facebook pages. A sense of real community – or was it shared grief and terror? – began to take hold. Someone set up a simple shrine to Jao Mae Nang Non, as the Sleeping Lady is known, and people began to leave offerings of soda, boiled eggs, fruit and desserts. No one could provide a spiritual explanation for why the Sleeping Lady might have decided to trap the boys in the cave. But the youngsters would be found, it was widely agreed, once she was fully satisfied. 'We all believe that all places have guardian spirits, places like mountains, caves and houses,' as one local woman explained. 'We may not see them, but they can see us. So we need to respect them when we go into their places.'

Tents were brought in for the distraught parents, who vowed to remain at the cave until their sons were found. As the rain kept falling, the tents were not nearly enough to keep anyone dry.

Over the next days, more military personnel arrived, including Royal Thai Navy SEALs, with offers of assistance now pouring in from Australia, China, Britain, Belgium, Scandinavia and America. A team of United States Air Force pararescuers were said to be coming. As the media horde continued to grow, Chiang Rai governor Narongsak Osottanakorn, who holds degrees in geology and engineering, took personal charge of the scene. There was still no clear rescue plan. But the straight-talking governor began to issue orders and hold regular briefings, and he brought some basic order to the chaos of the cave site. One of his first acts was to separate the families from the media.

'Whatever part you play in the mission,' he said to rescuers and responders at the scene, 'I ask you to think of the boys as your own children. That is how much we care about them. We won't abandon them. We are in this fully.'

As news of the boys' plight spread, the international cave-diving community was also springing into action. This was a tightly knit global fraternity, avid civilians mostly, men and women who pursued cave diving as a challenging adventure sport. The divers and their dry-caver friends also came together from time to time to rescue people who were lost inside flooded caves – or, more frequently, to recover the bodies of those who had perished there. Not surprisingly, the people closest to Tham Luang got there first. No one arrived sooner than Vern Unsworth, and the boys were so lucky he did.

A plain-spoken 63-year-old British caver and financial broker from the historic city of St Albans, Hertfordshire, Vern Unsworth had learned caving as a boy in the dales of Yorkshire. Now, he lived part of the year in Chiang Rai, an hour's drive south of the cave. He got a call the morning after the boys were lost and came right over. He'd spent years exploring the cave, tracing its narrow passages and blind turn-offs, taking notes and measurements, numbering the chambers and making himself thoroughly at home. He'd gone further and deeper than anyone before him. Having Vern there so quickly was a tremendous benefit. He spoke to Governor Osottanakorn and the other local officials. He warned some of the more gung-ho first responders about the dangers of thoughtlessly rushing in. He explained the layout of the cave and shared his personal maps. Vern even offered his best-guess prediction about where the boys would likely be found. He said he didn't think they'd have wandered into a part of the cave known as Monk's Series. 'It is not a very nice section,' he said. 'Most people go left and head for a section called Pattaya Beach.'

Pattaya Beach is a big sandbank, about two and a half kilometres in, named for Thailand's famous tourist beach.

'This isn't a job for normal cavers,' Vern told the Thai authorities in no uncertain terms. 'We need people with diving experience.'

Not the Thai Army or Navy. Not even the elite Thai Navy SEALs, who were trained in combat diving and maritime counter-terrorism but not in the special challenges of cave diving. The SEALs had plenty of heart, and they were trying their best in the cave. But they weren't used to squeezing their bodies through openings no wider than their hips or swimming through swirling water the colour of Caterers Blend coffee, let alone swimming beneath hundreds of metres of rock where there was no escape up to the surface if trouble appeared. Rescuing these children was a job for highly experienced specialists, Vern said, people like the veteran sump divers associated with the British Cave Rescue Council, adventurers who felt entirely at home in a constricted, low-visibility, underwater environment. The SEALs and other Thai troops could provide valuable support, Vern said. 'But this is a race against time. Only world-class divers will save these kids.'

Vern got some knowing nods. But by Tuesday afternoon, none of the Thai officials had acted on his pleas. The SEALs and others kept diving, but they hadn't found the boys. The rain had let up a bit, which was promising. But the sky was still cloudy, and no one could say when the next storm might blow in. As far as Vern was concerned, now was the last chance for action. It was literally do-or-die.

The SEALs were getting some help from a well-known cave diver who had also shown up at the scene. Ben Reymenants was his name. A 45-year-old Belgian who owned the Blue Label dive shop and diving school on the southern Thai resort island of Phuket, Ben was a media-savvy businessman-diver with a brash personal style. Harry and I knew Ben well. We'd been on a couple of diving trips with him, including one eighteen months earlier to Thailand's Song Hong, a sinkhole Ben had dived to about 180 metres. On that trip, we managed to push that out to the bottom at 196 metres. Only a very small number of people around the world specialise in this deep diving, and Ben is one of them.

Ben laid a considerable length of line inside Tham Luang cave in the early days of the mission, diving in very high water flow and very poor visibility, pushing the boundaries of what the less-experienced SEALs had been able to achieve. These were risky dives, as Ben recounted them in his interviews with journalists and his own frequent social-media reports. But it wasn't Ben Reymenants that Vern Unsworth touted to the increasingly anxious Thai officials. As it happened, while Vern had been assisting the early responders in a front part of the cave, he had received a call from a long-time caving partner who'd returned home to England from Thailand the week before. Vern's friend, Rob Harper, mentioned that he knew two of the greatest cave divers on earth. Those were the kinds of people Vern had in mind.

Around 9 p.m. on Tuesday, he was called into a meeting with Interior Minister Anupong Paochinda and Minister of Tourism and Sports Weerasak Kowsurat. The governor was also there, sitting quietly at the conference table. As the ministers reviewed the latest, fruitless efforts, Vern grabbed a pen and wrote a short note. He passed the note to the tourism-and-sports minister. The note read:

> Time is running out! 1) Rob Harper; 2) Rick Stanton MBE; 3) John Volanthen – they're the world's best cave divers. Please contact them through UK Embassy ASAP.

'What do you want me to do?' the minister asked after reading Vern's note, sounding like a man in an uncomfortable squeeze.

'What do you do?' Vern shot back. 'Call them now. Here's my phone.'

Rob Harper's contact was still open. But instead of pressing the WhatsApp phone icon, Vern mistakenly hit the one for video call. When Rob Harper answered, he sounded half-asleep. More-than-half asleep. Though it was midafternoon in England, he was in his pyjamas lying in bed. When the minister apologised, Rob explained that he was a veterinary surgeon who often worked at night. But he was fully awake now and eager to be helpful in Thailand any way he could.

The British Cave Rescue Council handled the logistics. Rob, Rick Stanton and John Volanthen were on the late-night flight from Heathrow to Bangkok. Finally, things were about to change.

When Rick, John and Rob arrived at the cave site, they went looking for Vern, who took them to meet the diving supervisor, a stern-faced Thai military officer stationed at the mouth of the cave. He was not especially welcoming to Rick and John. His men had been giving their all, taking risks they were not fully trained for, pushing themselves to the edge of exhaustion day and night. What could these two middle-aged hobbyists from Britain possibly achieve that his fit, young Navy special operators could not?

Rick and John were the most experienced cave divers on site by far. But they had no rank or authority. When the Thai military commander denied them access to the cave, the British divers were incensed. They'd dropped everything to show up in Thailand. Their skills and experience were obviously superior. And now they were being told they couldn't even enter the cave? Fortunately, the dispute worked its way quickly up to the top of the Ministry of Foreign Affairs. Late on Wednesday, word came down from the top SEAL commander, Rear Admiral Arpakorn Yuukongkaew.

'Just let them go.'

The Brits quickly gathered their gear and pushed past the throng of media outside the mouth of the cave. 'We've got a job to do' was all John would say as he and Rick brushed past the reporters who tried to question them. Finally, they were doing what they had come to do.

The initial dives through the first chambers were tough. Tougher than they expected. Strong, swirling rapids of dirty brown water made accurate navigation impossible. They pointed their noses into the strongest flow and groped their way forwards. Just reaching chamber 3, the large dry chamber that was to become the advanced staging post for future dives, was tremendously difficult. When they finally reached that point in the cave, they had their first shock.

For a brief moment on Thursday, Rick and John thought they might have found the boys. Rick heard a noise. It sounded like a rock being tossed and hitting the water. Following the sound, they were appalled to find themselves face to face with four Thai men in orange overalls, employees of the Thai Well Water Association, including association president Surapin Chaichompoo. The four Thai men had been part of a civilian work crew trying to pump water out of the cave. After hours of gruelling effort, the exhausted workers decided to take a nap in a quiet corner of chamber 3. When they woke, they were trapped by rising water. Everyone else had evacuated. No one seemed to notice these four had been left behind. The British divers had no choice but to temporarily abandon their search for the Wild Boars and rescue these members of what was clearly becoming an increasingly large and unwieldy cast of workers, engineers, soldiers, rescuers and volunteers.

Since the British divers shared no common language with the Thai labourers, Rick and John could use only hand signals to explain to the stranded men that, one at a time, they would be escorted through the ten-metre sump connecting chambers 3 and 2. The dive was shallow, but it was tight and made more so by the clutter of cables and pipes that had already been laid into the cave. Rick and John took turns, using each other's masks and cylinders as they began to shuffle the workers through.

On Monday, 2 July, nine days after the boys disappeared, Rick and John swam back into chamber 3. It was large enough and dry enough to become a combination warehouse, dorm room and forward operating base, an ideal spot from which to launch deeper explorations. Other divers, including the awesome lads from the Australian Federal Police, had been ferrying in air tanks and additional equipment. Military MREs – meals ready to eat – and cartons of bottled water had also been carried in, enough to sustain a long stay. Many of the Thai Navy SEALs brought in sleeping-bags and space blankets.

Rick Stanton and John Volanthen kept pressing forwards into the darkness, laying more line and searching each new section of cave for any signs of life. Every time they surfaced into an air space, they removed their masks and sniffed the air. If the boys were here, dead or alive, there would be some evidence of that, and smell is always one of the experienced divers' greatest assets. But they found nothing. Finally, they reached Pattaya Beach, the flat, sandy area where Vern had predicted the boys might be found. Rick and John surveyed the beach, from one end to the other. It looked like the kind of place that tired or frightened young explorers might set up camp. But there was no sign of the boys.

The divers continued on. But they didn't go much further. About 300 metres past Pattaya Beach, they reached an air space above the surface of the water, lifted their heads and removed their masks. They had a look. They sniffed the air. They still didn't see anything, but they sure smelled something. What was it? Excrement? Death? They fully expected to swim forwards through the long canal and bump into the floating bodies of the children. It was a chilling moment for the duo.

But then the light from John's helmet lamp revealed a truly exhilarating sight: up to the right, several boys were stepping out of the darkness, walking down a sloping path from a muddy ledge, directly towards them.

What a beautiful sight it was!

Rick started counting the boys. But before he could get to all of them, John called out in English: 'How many of you?'

'Thirteen!' came the reply, also in English.

'Thirteen? Brilliant!'

Just 300 metres from the spot where Vern had said they would be.

If John and Rick were excited to see Coach Ekk and the boys, the feeling was more than mutual. The Wild Boars were positively thrilled when the British divers appeared. This was the moment they'd been desperately waiting for, a moment some of them had begun to fear might never come. And now here it was. In their excitement, many of the boys seemed to assume they would all be leaving the cave that day. So there was a bit of a let-down when Rick and John had to explain that a swift departure wasn't possible. But they promised, as they wrapped up their short visit, that they and other divers would definitely be back soon.

Before saying goodbye, they left some lights and some energy bars with the boys, and they captured the brief encounter on John's helmet-mounted video camera. When the short video was posted on the Navy SEALs' Facebook page soon after they left the cave,

it was the first real piece of good news in nine exhausting, excruciating, emotionally draining days, and it didn't come a minute
too soon. Hope and celebration erupted at the cave site, where the
parents, classmates, rescuers and volunteers had grown so weary
they could barely stand it. Then, happiness for the boys spread
via the media all around the world, as some of the details of their
underground captivity began to leak out.

They'd been sleeping on the ledge where Rick and John had
found them without so much as a single blanket to keep them warm.
They'd been drinking the water that had flowed by them in the
cave. They'd been without food for nine long days. They'd been
wandering around a corner to relieve themselves. And yet in the
video, they all sounded remarkably cheerful. The boys and the coach
all flashed wonderful, happy smiles. They all looked healthy at first
glance. Could things really have gone so well for them in Tham
Luang cave? Rick and John could only report what they saw. And for
now it was encouraging.

They're alive!

The boys and their young coach are alive!

Now the hard work would begin.

Crucial and exhilarating though it was, the exciting discovery in the
cave was only a start.

It didn't mean the Wild Boars and Coach Ekk were out of Tham
Luang yet. It didn't mean they would ever see the light of day or their
families and friends again. It didn't mean they wouldn't die today or
tomorrow or next week or next month, two and a half kilometres
from the rest of their lives. The cave was still flooded. Its passages
were still narrow and treacherous. The boys and the coach still had

no diving experience. The sky outside was still menacing and dark. And time was ticking loudly for everyone.

The chances of a successful outcome were still extraordinarily slim. That was the frank assessment of anyone who knew, meaning anyone who had ever even considered the awesome responsibility of rescuing a human being stranded inside a flooded cave. As the days wore on, Harry and I were still exchanging emails, text messages and phone calls with many of the top cave divers in the world.

There was no hint of this pessimism in the relentless media coverage, which Harry and I kept devouring back home, itching for some way to play a role in the rescue and considering that prospect increasingly remote. The discovery of the boys was being hailed in the media as such a massive triumph, it felt almost rude to wonder out loud:

So what happens next?

Photos of the young players were everywhere, accompanied by their bare-bones biographies and their snappy nicknames. Mark. Mick. Pong. Tern. Titan. Here they were in their red, blue and black soccer jerseys. There they were in photos at school. Now, they're pictured with their precious families. Often, these fetching images were paired with snatches of painful interviews with their shell-shocked parents, who sounded exhilarated that the boys had been located but also devastated that no one seemed to know how to bring them home.

It was the perfect media narrative. High stakes. Cute kids. With the ultimate human question at its core: would they live or would they die? And here was the twist: the answer was in the hands of some middle-aged cave divers who looked nothing like any action heroes the media had ever seen before.

The story brought out the good in many people, including those who lived closest to the cave. Fresh volunteers kept appearing at the scene. Local women cooked hot noodles, chicken rice and other Thai delicacies. Even a couple of chefs from the Thai royal family pitched in. A hair stylist offered free cuts to anyone who was feeling shabby. Other volunteers cleaned the park's portable toilets and offered rides from the main road to the cave. An entire, instant town grew up with no real order or plan, just a lot of nice people trying to help, as the British were joined by a growing contingent of European divers and cavers, and the SEALs and Thai government officials got busy figuring out what to do next. Advice and ideas were pouring in from everywhere.

Giant pumps were moved into the front of the cave, their powerful sucking motors straining to reduce the water level. Engineers tried to calculate the best spots to drill an alternative exit from above, aiming to create a vertical tunnel the boys might climb out of or be lifted through somehow. Ben and the other diving instructors were constantly being asked if they could train a dozen eleven-to-sixteen-year-olds, none of whom had any scuba experience, to dive themselves out with tanks, masks and fins.

Nothing seemed especially promising except for the powerful pumps, which were pulling millions of litres of water out of the cave every hour. (How valuable that would be long term was still an open question.) But still, no ideas were rejected outright by the Thai authorities. How could anything be? No one could say for certain what might be the magic bullet here. And other ideas were percolating too. Elon Musk, the billionaire co-founder of PayPal whose next-generation tech firms included the automaker Tesla and space explorer SpaceX, was already making public inquiries about how his engineers might play a role. As these conversations continued, everyone kept looking up at the sky. Whichever schemes were ultimately adopted, they would all come to nothing if the rainfall resumed with a vengeance. The very best of intentions could all be washed away along with Coach Ekk and the dozen Wild Boars.

It was soon after Rick and John's big discovery that the Royal Thai Navy SEALs made an extraordinary offer. They would send in a seven-man team, some of whom would stay with the coach and the boys, watching over them and caring for them, as long as it took for a successful rescue to be achieved. The SEAL team would be led by a legendary Thai Army medic, Dr Pak Loharnshoon, known as Dr Pak, who had been through the full SEAL training course and was described by people who knew him as a talented, charismatic special-forces combatant and doctor. He too was said to have agreed: he would dive into chamber 9 with the SEALs, treat the boys as well as he was able to under these sparse conditions and remain with them however long it took to free them. With a few diving tips from Rick and John, Pak and the SEALs got up early the next morning and made what was for them an excruciating six-hour dive.

They found the water uncomfortably chilly. Several suffered from cramps along the way and had to rest. And the SEALs managed to consume most of the air in their tanks. They'd have to figure out later how to get the air they'd need to dive everyone out. It was nearly noon by the time the seven-man team arrived at chamber 9.

It turned out there was sufficient air for only three of the SEALs to dive out that day, leaving Pak and three others behind. But Pak and those three promised to stay with the boys as long as it took. 'Everyone can be relieved now, as the boys are in the good hands of Navy SEALs, who will be with them and take care of them all the time,' the commander told the media. 'It may be four months, one month or one week. There is no need to hurry. Safety is the priority. There will be constant food and medicine provided to the trapped footballers and a communication line to the outside world.'

The communication line would prove harder to establish than the commander imagined. What communicating occurred would be conducted the old-fashioned way, by divers carrying messages back and forth. The British divers had taken in further supplies: lights and batteries. Meals ready-to-eat from the US Air Force Pararescue team. But the SEAL team brought something else the players had been living without – outside companionship.

Now, the boys had the greatest babysitters ever!

5

Cave Chaos

Harry

As all this was unfolding in Thailand, I was home in Australia, trading text messages with Rick Stanton and Ben Reymenants at the scene. Rob Harper had to depart for a medical appointment back home in England. But other British and European divers were said to be on the way.

And what were Craig and I feeling back home in Australia?

Three things, actually. We were deeply relieved to know that the boys had been located by Rick and diving partner John Volanthen and were being cared for by the SEALs. We were just as deeply concerned that bringing the lads out safely still seemed to be such a terrible long shot. And we couldn't believe that this whole thing was happening without us being there. We *belonged* in Thailand. We knew we did. We'd just been angling for the right invitation.

It wasn't like we weren't getting any encouragement so far.

*

The possibility of our going kept being dangled in front of our eyes, beginning as early as 27 June, four days after the team members disappeared. That Wednesday morning, I got an email from Al Warild, a renowned caver from the east coast of Australia who is captain of the New South Wales Cave Rescue Squad. Al had spent nearly sixty years exploring some of the world's most challenging holes in the ground – in New Zealand, Mexico, Papua New Guinea and elsewhere – often solo and with very little equipment. His book, *Vertical*, is a real caver's bible. Now, Al wrote, he'd been asked by the Australian government to 'chase up cave divers' who could help in Thailand. 'Any ideas? Are you available? Know anyone suitable?'

I answered promptly. 'Craig and I could be available . . . Is it a recovery or a rescue?' No one knew at that point, five days before the boys were found, and that's the first question you've always got to ask. It turned out that, as Al was sounding me out, he was also firing off emails and a phone call to Western Australia, recruiting Craig. 'Craig is ok to go,' Al told me.

As we waited to hear more from Al, I got a message later that Wednesday from Ben, who sounded like he was in the middle of everything. A big crowd was gathering, he said, and he was making his way swiftly into the cave.

'Any excuse to pop over, mate!' I nudged him.

Ben answered noncommittally. 'Thanks, I'll let you know. Still raining, water is muddy and rising.'

I heard from Ben again Wednesday night:

I have two Thai guys that went in. Rick Stanton and 2 other British cave explorers arrived. Thai navy is pumping out water and trying to divert a waterfall which fills up the cave, but there's a very tight restriction the divers can't get past with their back mount, so it's side mount only. Focus is now on getting someone in to check if they're alive and sending supplies until the water drops.

The big news there, as far as I was concerned, was that Rick Stanton was on the scene. It was probably inevitable that Ben and Rick would eventually clash. If Rick and his British dive partners were involved, the rescue operation was almost certain to become more professional, pronto. Wherever Rick turns up, he tends to be followed by a trail of accolades. *The greatest . . . the most respected . . . the most experienced.* He has often been called 'the best cave diver in Europe', though most other cave divers would argue with that. 'What do you mean Europe?' they would add insistently. 'Why stop there? Rick's the best anywhere.' Rick had been involved in more rescues and body recoveries than most. Put it like this: if you're stuck in a cave, you want him on the scene – and not just because of the diving records he holds. He's at least as proud of his 'Hero of the Year' awards from the West Midland Fire Service. A firefighter for twenty-five years, he has the skills to make a difference and rescue is in his blood. If he could make a difference for the stranded Wild Boars, the 57-year-old diver would surely be hailed a hero again. But I also sensed an imminent clash between Rick and Ben. Two strong personalities. International legend versus local hotshot. Both of them now at Tham Luang cave.

Ben wrote to me again on Thursday morning:

Unsure what happened with Rick. But they went in the cave, had a huge discussion with the SEAL team and came out. Then I was called, so heading over there. Will keep you posted if

I need help. Unsure how to transport 12 kids over 1km distance in zero viz against flow. They can't swim and never dove.

The *can't swim* part would turn out later not to be true, but that was definitely the prevailing assumption at the time. Sitting back at home in Adelaide, it was hard to grasp all the undercurrents in Ben's texts – and I don't just mean the liquid kind. I got the feeling there was a Ben-team and a Rick-team, and they were working independently. But I was happy to keep up the dialogue with Ben. 'Give a call if you want to chat,' I wrote back to him. 'We have done some practice like this with FFMs, switch blocks and QDs' – full-face masks and devices for switching between different gas supplies.

At the same time, I had also reached out to Rick and John, offering encouragement and reminding them how willing Craig and I were to assist. 'Hi guys,' I wrote,

stay safe over there. I feel like I should be over there helping. If you manage to get to these guys, they will likely need medical assistance and you will need a team of divers to take turns to baby sit them while an extraction plan comes together, which may take some time. Craig and I are happy to provide any assistance to your team if required. All the best, Harry.

Barely an hour later, I heard back from Rick. 'Thanks for the offer of help,' he wrote. 'You've thought of the issues involved. Struggling to progress against the current and water unlikely to recede until end of monsoon season.'

'Bugger,' I answered. 'All sounds v sad.'

'Above statement best kept in relative confidence until the news is slowly released,' Rick cautioned, already noticing that the media coverage sounded far more optimistic than things were looking on the ground. 'There may still be other successful options in the meantime.'

The increasing free-for-all at the cave site – too many people, too little organisation, too much media – was undermining the mission, Rick said. 'We're pulling out as there's nothing we can do,' he wrote in his latest message to me. 'There's too many lies, false hopes and chaos. The military will take over the operation and continue to dive.'

'Oh dear,' I wrote back. 'Awful.' I hated the idea that a clash between divers could undermine the chance of the mission's success. 'You must feel like shit,' I wrote to Rick. 'Great you were there to try.'

'We're here maintaining a presence to present a positive image that all is well,' Rick said.

'Hope you can still contribute somehow,' I wrote, trying to be encouraging.

'The circus here is so large and chaotic most have lost track of purpose,' Rick answered.

'At least you saved some rescuers,' I said, saying all I could think of to sound consoling. I asked about the possibility of alternative entrances to the cave.

'Not much chance but certainly worth pursuing,' Rick answered.

'Poor buggers.'

'Yes.'

'I feel v sad,' I wrote. 'Can't imagine how you guys must feel.'

'We think the likely scenario is they fled a flood from the southern passage where they were headed,' he wrote, his mind still on search and rescue despite it all. 'Encountered a sump at Monks junction halting their exit. Then it's whether they were able to retreat back upstream to possible sanctuary at Pattaya beach, I suspect not as there are u bends that would fill.'

'Might be kinder if they couldn't escape it,' I wrote, raising a horrible but unavoidable possibility. This was how low everything had sunk.

'I agree,' Rick answered. 'Vern our local expert, who's been correct in every step of the flooding process we have observed, says it may not be until Dec or Jan until you can enter without some diving. i.e. the u bends will have drained.

'Yuck.'

And that, right there, could have been the end of it all. The Thai military, with almost no cave-diving experience, could have taken over all future efforts to locate and rescue the boys with whatever help they could get from Ben. Craig and I could have gone off on our long-planned cave-diving adventure amid the barren beauty of the Nullarbor Plain. And Rick Stanton, the greatest and most respected cave diver on earth, could have packed up his guys and his gear and grabbed the next flight from Bangkok to Heathrow.

The whole world is extremely fortunate the scenario did not unfold like that, no one more so than twelve junior soccer players and their young assistant coach, huddled somewhere in the darkness of Tham Luang cave. When I heard back from Rick on Sunday afternoon, the crisis at the cave site seemed to have been averted – *for now.*

Rick said things were starting to gel:

JV and I reached the Monks junction so there is now 800m of continuous rope beyond 3rd chamber. 500m to reach Pattaya beach from there. Much more airspaces than expected so passage beyond 350m is mainly canals with many short dives. Water dropping, 2 m Vis. We have a two day window to achieve something.

I didn't even ask Rick to explain the dramatic turn-around, I was so happy to receive the report. 'Great news,' I answered. 'I really wish I could be there in case they are alive and need medical attention.'

'They have Special Forces doctors ready to dive in on LAR rebreathers and live 3 months in the cave,' Rick said, the first I heard anything about Thai military personnel moving into the cave with the boys. 'The supply chain is unbelievably massive with many hundreds of Ali 80s going in,' referring to the common type of scuba cylinders used by divers. Then, Rick added the usual and necessary caveat: 'Needless to say this could all go very wrong when it rains. This is beyond our level, we're here as pathfinders.'

'Ah, ok,' I answered. 'Glad they have a plan. Keen to use my skills!'

It was the next afternoon, Monday, when Rick and John showed just how driven and talented they were, finally locating the Wild Boars on a muddy ledge just past Pattaya Beach. Interestingly, it was Ben who first called me with the news. Maybe peace really was breaking out at Tham Luang.

I texted my congratulations straight to Rick: 'Kids all alive! Wonderful news and congratulations!' By the next day, six Thai Navy SEALs, led by Thai Army doctor Pak Loharnshoon, had made the arduous dive in, with Pak and three others vowing to remain with the boys and the coach as long as it took to get everyone out.

All that sent a blast of optimism throughout the cave site, across Thailand and around the world. As far as the media were concerned, now that the boys had been located, the rest was just a matter of wrapping things up. *Hasn't the real work been accomplished? How hard could it be at this point to pull the young people out? Aren't they just sitting there?* I knew from our text messages and from all my years diving in caves that exactly the opposite was likely to be true. However hard finding them in the cave had been, getting them out of there was by far the bigger challenge.

'Hi Rick,' I wrote first thing on Wednesday morning, 'wondering if you are still on site. Would be great to get an update if you have any down time. Congrats again to you and John for the breakthrough. Fingers crossed for the next bit.'

'Will call you sometime,' Rick answered. He was already thinking about the next step. 'There's stuff to talk about. They are not being dived out by Thai navy. Could you sedate someone and dive them out ??'

That text was the first time Rick mentioned sedation to me. He couldn't be serious about that, I thought. *Diving a sedated child underwater? Through the twists and turns and narrow constrictions of a remote flooded cave?* I brushed past the notion with just a few words. 'Really?' I wrote back. 'What do you think about diving them out? Sedation not an option.' As for Craig and me, hope was fading quickly that we'd be on a plane for Thailand to help with the rescue. Time was running out. 'I would still come if you thought I could help,' I said to Rick. 'Leaving for Nullarbor in 24 hrs though.'

The window was closing quickly. It was about to slam shut.

When I got Craig on the phone, we agreed we should accept the inevitable and turn our attention to our own upcoming cave adventure on the Nullarbor Plain, which we'd been very excited about before Thailand came up. *Nullarbor* is Latin (*nullus arbor*) for 'no trees', and that's exactly what's there, 200,000 square kilometres of rugged, tree-less territory potholed with some utterly awe-inspiring caves. We'd be camping out of range of wi-fi or phone service. From the Nullarbor, we'd never be able to stay in touch with Rick and the guys in Thailand.

'Harry,' Craig said to me with a long sigh as we packed our trucks for the long drives the next morning, 'one of these days we will be involved in a great cave rescue. But this won't be the one.'

Much as I hated to, I had to concede that Craig was right.

In the two days since Rick and John had reached the boys, I could sense that the British divers were being afforded a whole new level of trust and respect around the cave site and across the diving world. Ben hadn't found the boys. The Thai Navy SEALs hadn't found the boys. The boys hadn't walked out on their own. Rick and John had found them. And soon, I suspected, they and their arriving British colleagues would gain more influence over the rescue-planning process.

By now, there was no shortage of rescue ideas floating around. Tham Luang was crawling with so-called experts, every one of whom seemed to have an opinion about how best to rescue the Wild Boar soccer boys. Pretty much anyone with a Twitter account was weighing in from around the world. From our text exchanges, I could tell that Rick and John didn't have any more confidence in most of these schemes than Craig or I did. That the cave could be effectively drained now that the rainy season had started. That the mountain drillers could aim perfectly enough to drill a hole to the exact spot where the boys were. Rick wasn't saying any of that was impossible, just that it shouldn't be counted on.

Perhaps the most striking ideas – others called them the most outlandish – came from tech billionaire Elon Musk. On Wednesday, the South African-born Musk announced on Twitter that he was 'happy to help' rescue the boys in Thailand, adding that he had ordered his top engineers to come up with a creative plan. They'd hatched several, it seemed.

The first was a nylon tube that could be inflated like a birthday-party bouncy castle to create an underwater air tunnel. The kids, he said, could then walk out of the cave, high and dry, without needing to dive at all. When divers on the scene noted that there was no way Elon's inflatable tunnel could even be transported through the cave passage, let alone survive the sharp rocks and narrow openings of the cave, he had another proposal.

A 'kid-size submarine'.

The minisub, he said, would be made from a Falcon 9 liquid oxygen transfer tube, large enough to hold a boy or two. He said he would begin testing the vessel in the swimming pool at Palisades Charter High School in Los Angeles straightaway and would person-ally deliver the sub to Thailand.

The details quickly leaked out: The sealed tube, 1.5 metres by 300 millimetres and weighing about 41 kilograms, would be propelled manually by divers in the front and back. In case the minisub could not fit through the narrow openings of the cave, Musk also asked the engineers at Wing Inflatables, a California-based inflat-able boat manufacturer, to build blow-up escape pods. The pods were designed, fabricated and tested in one day before being flown to Thailand.

It is fair to say that no prominent cave divers or anyone who knew much about caves greeted Musk's ideas with much enthusiasm. But hey, who knew? All contributions were welcome, right?

Rick, Craig, John and I were equally sceptical of another idea that seemed to be gaining some currency: just leave the boys inside. Wait for the rainy season to end. Let the water drain from the cave, as it did most years by December. Supply the young people with food and water and other necessities until they could be safely walked out. As someone intimately familiar with the challenging environments of flooded caves, Rick didn't trust any of that. As a cave-diving doctor, I thought the idea was nuts. Trying to sustain thirteen young people deep inside a cave for months on end would be a medical nightmare. What would happen when they started getting dysentery? How would the site stay clean? Where would they go to the toilet? How would you keep them dry and warm? What would you do with all the dead bodies, as the boys succumbed one at a time? The issues were insurmountable. In Rick's mind – and in mine – you'd only be replacing a fast death with a slow one.

Then, there was the idea of outfitting the team members with tanks, regulators, masks, fins and wetsuits and, after some brief instruction, diving them out. It sounded nice. But all of us doubted the notion that a crash scuba course could prepare a dozen boys and their young coach for such a challenging underwater environment. Hadn't it just taken a team of exceptional Navy SEALs six gruelling hours to dive *in*? The SEALs were fit, military special operators with years of diving experience – not a soccer team of eleven-to-sixteen-year-olds.

But as we all weighed these various options and found each of them profoundly unpromising in one way or another, Rick kept returning to some questions he was obviously wrestling with. *What if the young people were unconscious? What if they didn't have any idea what was happening to them? What if they were under the blanket of a powerful drug?*

I understood why Rick was drawn to sedation. It answered one of the stronger objections to diving the boys out the conventional way. An inexperienced young person, under water for a long time in such a hostile environment, would almost certainly panic at some point. Panic is a powerful human reflex, nearly impossible to control. On a long underwater journey, it could easily be deadly, accompanied by violent movement, flailing arms, the yanking of hoses and face masks – and goodness knows what else. That panic could easily kill the boys and possibly even the expert divers escorting them.

'You've sedated thousands of patients over the years, young and old,' Rick said to me at one point.

I told him I had. 'In hospitals and sometimes at accident sites on the side of a road. But never in a cave. Never once in a cave.'

Sedating these children, I emphasised to Rick, would entail a bevy of other unique risks, starting with the most basic one: how on earth could you dive unconscious children through a long and dangerous cave without drowning them? Diving requires the active participation of the diver. What happens when water leaks into the face mask? What happens when an air hose fails? How would you know what dose to administer? What would you do when the drug wore off? To me, diving while sedated sounded almost as reckless as leaving the boys inside the cave.

But Rick kept raising this novel idea. And he kept reminding me: we weren't hunting for the perfect solution, only the best one.

'What's better than this?' he asked.

I have heard people say that it's darkest just before the dawn. Strictly speaking, I don't believe that's true. I've been up at that hour quite a few times. As dawn approaches, the sky gets brighter, not darker. And that's exactly what happened here. I sent one last message to Rick Stanton before Craig and I headed off the grid. Little did I expect, that would be the message that landed.

'Craig and I are happy to come and help,' I reminded Rick for about the ten-thousandth time. 'I don't know if there's anything specifically we can do, but if you feel like there's a need for a couple of extra pairs of hands, people you know and trust, we'll come.'

'I think we could use you,' Rick said finally. 'And if the issue of sedation doesn't go away, you're the guys to do it.'

Craig and I were going to Thailand at last.

II

Going

6

Home Front

Harry

You can't just show up in Thailand and start rescuing a bunch of stranded children, even if Rick Stanton asks you to come. This is the twenty-first century. Procedures must be followed, and approvals obtained. It was no longer possible to sneak in and out of Tham Luang cave, as it had been in the early days, not with an occupying army of rescuers, government officials, media people and volunteers crowded nearby. This was not the equivalent of Craig and me slipping into an out-of-the-way cave somewhere for a sneaky dive without asking the owner's permission. I'm not saying we've done that before, but it'd be possible, I'm sure. This time, millions of people were watching around the world.

'So how do we make this happen?' I asked Rick. 'Are there any Australian government people on the ground there?' I thought things might go more smoothly if my government coordinated with the Thai government in some official way. Governments deal with governments every day, don't they? Isn't that what diplomacy is all about?

'Yeah, some Australians are here,' Rick said. 'Federal police and some diplomatic people.'

That was a start, at least. 'Could you just chat with them and tell them you've spoken to me?' I said to Rick. 'Say I'm happy to come, and could they start the ball rolling? Because I wouldn't have a clue who to call in Australia.'

Rick promised to try.

Within an hour, I got a call from Canberra. The man on the phone said he was from DFAT, the Department of Foreign Affairs and Trade. 'Dr Harris?' he said. 'We'd like you to go to Thailand, and I'm here to facilitate that.'

Wow, that was easy! Rick had delivered! He'd even made it seem like it was Canberra's idea!

The man on the phone said that AUSMAT – the Australian Medical Assistance Team – would be taking part in an official mission authorised by DFAT. (Yes, everything goes by initials in Canberra.) AUSMAT members are called upon by various state and federal government bodies to provide medical aid after major disasters at home and overseas. If there's an earthquake somewhere like Papua New Guinea, a team of doctors, nurses and logistics people will be airlifted in to support relief and recovery efforts. Usually, these teams are large. Many people. Diverse skills. Massive containers filled with equipment and supplies, up to and including full field hospitals.

I had taken the AUSMAT training courses and was already on the books as an AUSMAT doctor, though I had never actually been deployed on a mission. But they knew of me, and apparently that made things easier from a bureaucratic point of view. I was pre-vetted, a known quantity.

'The simplest way for us to do this is to send you over as an AUSMAT representative, a team of one,' I was told. 'You'll be a

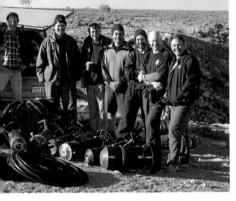
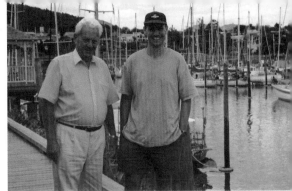

Top left: L-R: Geoff Paynter, Richard Harris, Ken Smith, Craig Challen, John Currie, Simon Doughty and Mark Brown. At the finish of the 2008 Cocklebiddy expedition after extending the known cave for the first time since 1995. *Photo by Geoff Paynter*

Top right: Harry with his father, James Dunbar Harris, in Whangarei, New Zealand, in 1997.

On our expedition with the Wet Mules diving group in China. Behind Harry and Craig lies the Daxing Spring, which the team dived to 213m depth. *Photo by Heather Endall*

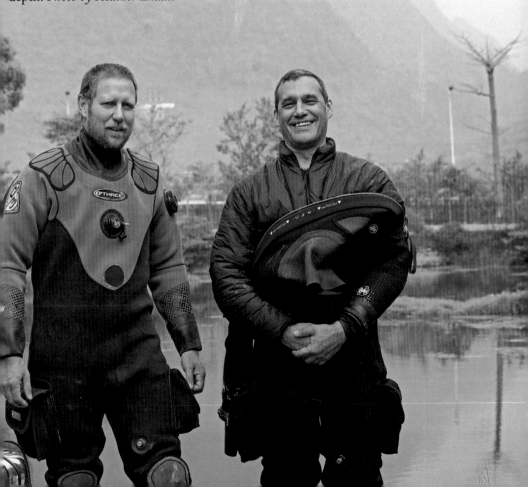

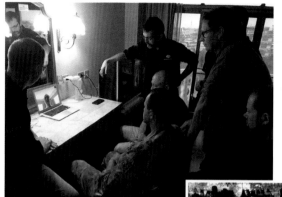

Shortly after everyone was safely out of the cave successfully, Prime Minister Malcolm Turnbull spoke to the Australian rescuers on a Skype call, which was set up in a tiny hotel room.

Our interpreter, Kittanu Supasamsen, or Nu for short. Nu's job usually involved getting rowdy Australians out of jail, so the cave rescue was a new adventure for him.
Photo by Richard Harris

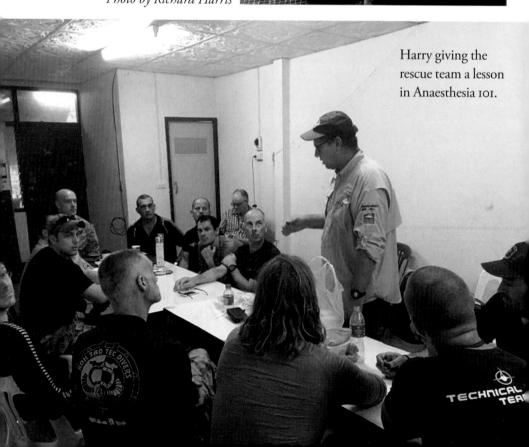

Harry giving the rescue team a lesson in Anaesthesia 101.

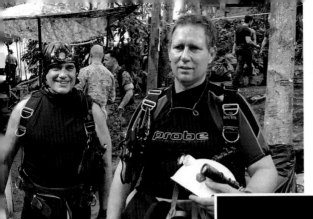

Craig and Harry back at the surface after a day in the cave.

Craig in the ambulance during the 'escape' from meeting the Thai prime minister, accompanied by Kittanu and the Thai medical and nursing staff.

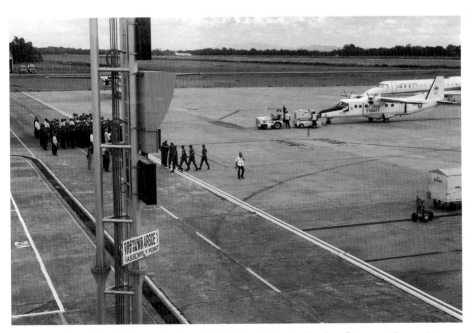

As Harry disembarks from the plane in Chiang Rai, the body of Saman Gunan is loaded into the Thai Navy aircraft on the right. A military parade gives Saman a send-off. *Photo by Richard Harris*

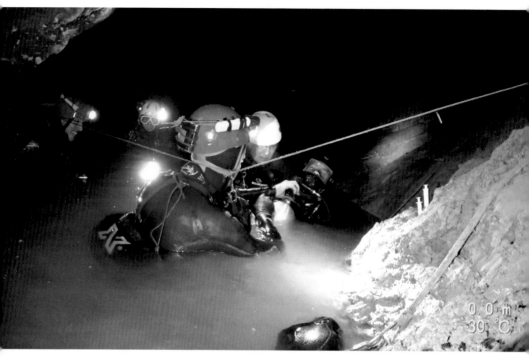

Above: The boy is asleep, his full face mask is on and Chris Jewell is strapping the cylinder to his chest. In the background, Rick and John await their turns. *Photo by Richard Harris. Below:* A syringe was used to anaesthetise the boys and the coach in order for us to safely perform the rescue. *Photo by Josh Morris*

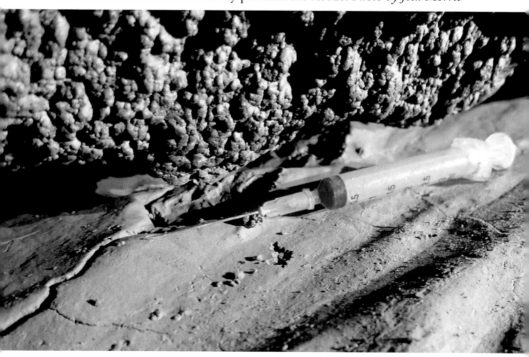

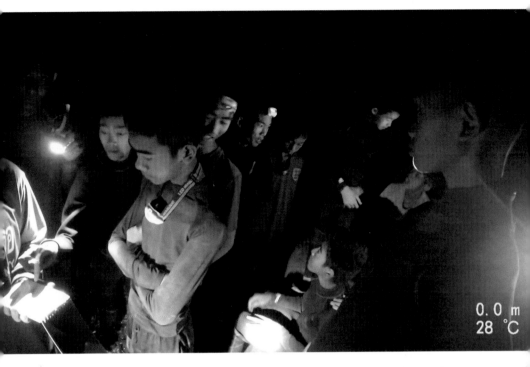

Above: At the top of the steep slope in chamber 9, the boys await their turn to escape the cave. *Below:* Only their lights can be seen. On the slope itself Dr Pak (rear) and a Navy SEAL chat with Harry.

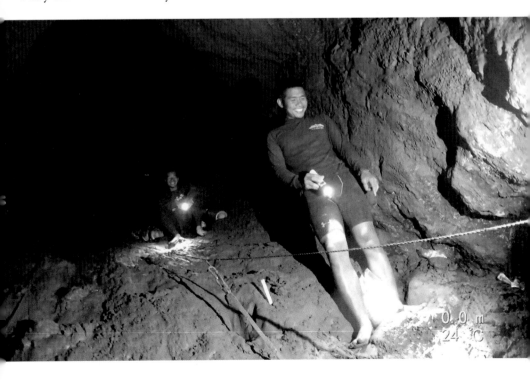

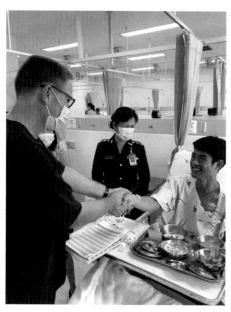
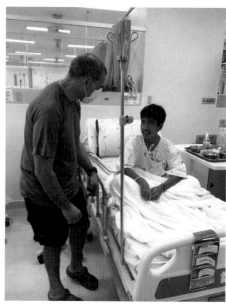

Above: Harry greeting Coach Ekk (left) and Craig with one of the older boys (right) in the hospital after the successful rescue mission.

Below: Meeting young Titan in the hospital after the rescue. Always smiling!

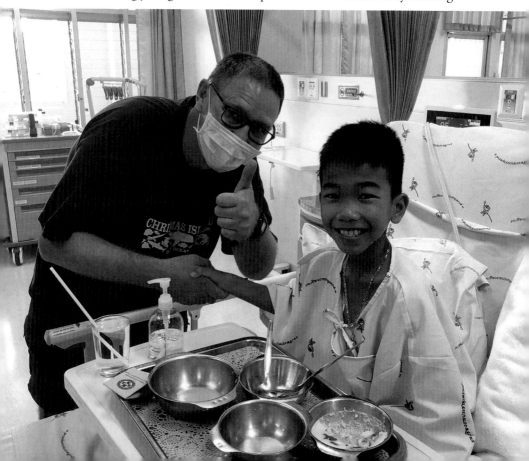

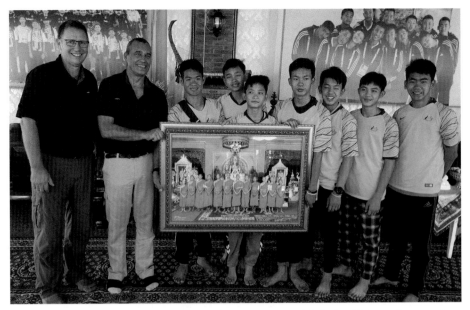

Nine months after the rescue, Craig and Harry visit six of the Wild Boars boys and Coach Ekk at a temple in Thailand.

Reunited with two of their rescuers, the boys take turns kneeling in front of Craig and Harry, bowing and resting their head a moment on the divers' knees, before getting up and sharing a hug.

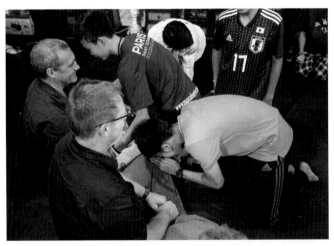

John Volanthen, Rick Stanton and Craig relax at Le Méridien Chiang Rai resort. *Photo by Richard Harris*

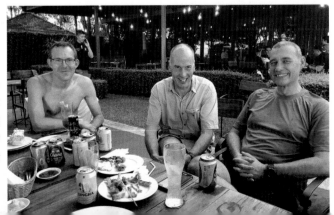

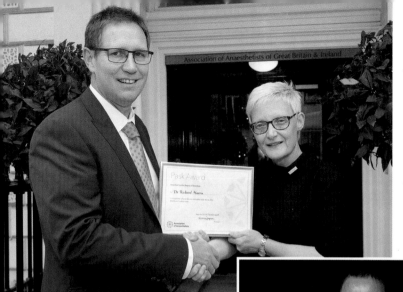

An honour: Harry receiving the Edgar Pask Citation from Dr Kathleen Ferguson on behalf of the Association of Anaesthetists of Great Britain and Ireland in London, December 2018.

Craig and Harry after being awarded Australians of the Year 2019. *Photo by Mick Tsikas/AAP*

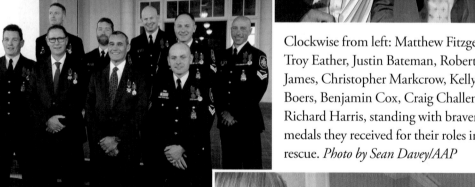

Clockwise from left: Matthew Fitzgerald, Troy Eather, Justin Bateman, Robert James, Christopher Markcrow, Kelly Boers, Benjamin Cox, Craig Challen and Richard Harris, standing with bravery medals they received for their roles in the rescue. *Photo by Sean Davey/AAP*

Harry and Craig meeting Their Royal Highnesses the Duke and Duchess of Sussex at Admiralty House during their Royal Tour of Australia. *Photo courtesy Government House* government employee. You'll report to the Australian government through a DFAT person on the ground.'

Personally, I didn't care who authorised the trip – I'd be happy to represent the Australian darts team – just as long as the trip was approved. But before I agreed to go anywhere, I had to get something straight.

Team of one? How about a team of two?

'This is important,' I said to the man from Canberra. 'I need this bloke called Craig Challen to come with me. He's my dive buddy.'

That was greeted with silence on the line.

'Um,' the man said with a sigh. 'That could be an issue.'

'If I'm going to do this,' I insisted, 'I need a trusted ally in the water with me – and more importantly, on the surface, to help me argue through everything. He's a highly experienced diver. I need Craig there.'

It was then patiently explained to me that, whatever Dr Challen's particular talents, he was not a member of AUSMAT. There was no quick and easy way to approve his joining the mission. 'I'm sorry,' the man said.

'I'm sorry,' I said. 'Let me put it another way: if he doesn't go, I don't go.'

I wasn't bluffing. When there's a complex diving problem, Craig and I can always tease things out together. He'll challenge my assumptions. He'll think of things I didn't think of. Just explaining my thinking to Craig forces a certain rigour on me. And it's mutual. I do the same for him. I couldn't imagine a mission much more complex than this one. I needed my trusted arguer at my side. We had a lot to thrash out here. Young lives were at stake. We had to make sure we weren't doing anything dumb.

I had no trouble imagining the nightmare scenarios. On the Agnes recovery, we had found that if you're the one who's handling the body, it's very hard to look after your air consumption, to navigate and to think about all the other things you need to consider at the same time. That time, we had a system in place. One guy was in charge of looking after Ag, and the other guy was in charge of keeping us both safe. Each situation is different, but I knew Craig would always have my back underwater if my head was in another place dealing with these kids.

'I know Craig's a guy who's not going to crumble under pressure,' I said. 'He won't get disturbed by whatever is going on around us, even if that means bringing dead children out of the cave. Craig will be all right.'

'Hmm . . .' That's all I got on the other end of the line.

Then the questions began, which I took as a hopeful sign.

'Who is he again?'

'Craig Challen,' I said. 'He's a vet, a retired vet.'

'Was he involved in the government in any way?'

Some quick thinking: 'We did a rope rescue course together once, and he was going to do some work with the firemen from Urban Search and Rescue in WA,' I said. 'So yeah, I think he's in USAR in Western Australia.'

I didn't know that for sure. In fact, I was pretty sure I had just told a fib. Was that wrong? I was just giving the man something to hang his hat on. But it seemed to work. 'Good, good,' he said. 'He's in the government. We'll get onto it.'

That didn't fully seal the deal, I understood. But it did finally get things pointed the right way. I got a call later with more questions: 'We can't really find any record of him,' the man said. 'It's all very tricky. Are you sure you need him?'

'Yes,' I declared again. 'I'm not going without him.'

'Let's see what we can do.' And that was the strongest encourage-ment I got.

I wasn't sure why this request threw Canberra into such a spin, but it had definitely made everyone uncomfortable. They seemed to take my request seriously, though, and they threw lots of people and resources at vetting Craig – pardon the pun – and getting all his paperwork sorted out.

'Is he all right to send to Thailand?' I was asked.

'Yes.'

'Is he going to die, or sue us?'

'No.'

'He might have to indemnify us, just in case.'

'Okay.'

In the end, that was pretty much it. Both of us were good to go. Both of us. I shot off a message to Rick: 'We are on way. Arrive about lunchtime tomorrow.'

'Excellent,' Rick wrote back immediately.

So instead of contemplating the sixteen-hour drive to meet Craig for our Australian dive trip, I was pulling gear out of the truck, everything we would have needed for a week in a place as desolate as the Nullarbor Plain. The steaks and the beer had to come out of the truck fridge and into the kitchen fridge. The tanks had to go back in my shed. I would bring my mask and my regula-tors and a few other bits and pieces to Thailand. From what Rick had told me, the front part of the cave was already looking like a dive-shop warehouse, air tanks stacked high against the walls. As I unpacked, the phone was ringing so constantly that Fiona had to answer the calls.

I didn't really have to tell anyone at work I was on my way.

They had just assumed I was going, even before I was. For days, people had been saying: 'Oh, I thought you'd be in Thailand by now.'

At home in Gnangara outside Perth, Craig had been discussing all of this with Heather. Not surprisingly, she had some feelings on the subject.

'I don't want you to go,' she said.

Heather had been gripped by the TV coverage of the boys in the cave, even more so once the possibility arose that Craig might actually play a role in rescuing them. She has two grown boys of her own, and she could empathise deeply with the mums. But she had been hearing snippets of Craig's conversations with me and the other divers, and that gave her cause for concern.

'There's so much turmoil over there,' she said to Craig. 'It sounds like anarchy. There are all these people, and nobody knows what's going on. It's wonderful they found the boys, but I don't like the way any of the rest of it sounds.'

Craig and Heather are both independent, strong-willed people. They have what I would describe as a very frank relationship. Neither one of them hesitates to speak up. Not for a second did Heather doubt Craig's skill or experience. She knew he was a highly capable diver. And from what she'd heard about the inside of Tham Luang cave, it didn't sound nearly as dangerous as dive sites like the Pearse Resurgence, which she had always found terrifying. It was more the scene around the cave.

'It'll be chaos there,' Heather said. 'I know you. You'll be frustrated or reckless. One or the other. Neither one of those is good.'

Craig listened. Then he answered exactly as I would have expected him to. 'I'm going,' he said. 'Of course I'm going. What are you talking about?'

Heather wasn't giving up just like that, also as expected. 'Craig,' she said, 'have you really thought about this?' The boys had already been found, she reminded him. So he wasn't needed for that. And so much could still go wrong. 'How does it play in your head, the pressure of having the world watching this story?' she asked. 'People die. You know how it is in the diving fraternity. You meet someone at a dive conference or on a trip or out for dinner. Then you hear that person is dead. It's like – yeah? This won't be like any other dive. The eyes of the world will be on you.'

Craig heard Heather out. He knew she was speaking from genuine concern. 'Of course I'm going,' he said. 'Can you take me to the airport, please?'

Heather said, sure, she'd drive him to the airport in Perth.

Before I finished packing, I called my dad. Just three weeks earlier he'd moved into a nursing home. Nursing homes were not a good subject in our family. When my mother reached her early seventies, she had begun to lose her memory. As she slipped into dementia, the cranky part of her personality came to the fore. She had a fall, broke a bone in her back and spent a couple of weeks in the hospital. It soon became obvious that Dad wasn't going to be able to care for her at home. She spent the final four years of her life at the Regis Burnside nursing home in the Adelaide suburb of Linden Park, disappearing into her little sparrow of a body, finally slipping away. The carers were terrific, but the facility seemed dreary and old. Dad visited every day, unless he knew that one of my sisters or I was stopping by to see her. He was the most devoted husband imaginable. My mum's death tore him apart. The whole experience left the family exhausted and sad.

A year before my mother died, my father was diagnosed with a rare oesophageal cancer. It was a nasty, aggressive one. I went with him to see the oncologist, who said grimly: 'Well, Jim, if you don't have any treatment, I reckon it will be about six months. If you have chemotherapy and some radiotherapy, it might be about a year.'

Hmm . . .

Dad had always been keen on euthanasia. For twenty years, he'd been explicit about his end-of-life wishes. 'I don't want to be doing any of that chemo or horrible surgery at the end,' he told Amanda, Kristina and me. 'When my time comes, I'll be ready to go.'

But sitting in the oncologist's office that morning, I couldn't believe what came out of my father's mouth: 'All right, then,' he said. 'Let's do everything.'

What?

I told the oncologist: 'We'll go away and have a chat with the family. We'll come back and let you know.'

As my father and I walked out to the car, I spoke up. 'Dad, where on earth did that come from? Do everything? That's the last thing you've been telling us you want.'

He thought about it some more and talked it over with the family and rapidly settled on a far more modest course. He and I went back to the doctor, and I explained what had been discussed. 'What about a little bit of focused radiotherapy? A couple of zaps so he doesn't get swallowing problems.'

Well, bugger me, it bloody cured him!

One course of radiotherapy, and the tumour in my father's oesophagus seemed to completely disappear. We started calling him 'The Faker'. He wasn't actually cured, of course. He had an enlarged lymph node that kept growing. But he had no other serious symptoms for the next two and a half years. My father was given one of the most precious gifts of all, the gift of unexpected healthy time. He'd already lived four decades longer than his father and uncle. Out of the blue, he was handed another round of bonus time!

His mates took him fishing – on a very large boat, because he wasn't so steady on his feet any more. The fishing was slow that day. But one of his friends had brought along some frozen fillets of fish in a plastic bag. While my father was pouring himself another drink, the friend hooked the bag on my dad's line and called out excitedly: 'Jim! Your rod! Your rod!'

My father rushed back and grabbed his rod and reel. He gave the reel a few frantic spins, quickly pulling in the line. And there, dangling from the hook for everyone to see, was a plastic bag of frozen fish fillets.

No one loved a surprise more than my father did, and he roared with laughter.

But in early May, he had a serious fall. He spent two weeks in St Andrew's Hospital. By then, he was having short-term memory problems. He'd stopped driving and was feeling trapped in the house. Amanda and Kristina were especially attentive, helping with meals, bringing him the newspapers, dropping in to see him every day, sometimes twice a day.

After Mum's experience, he'd often said to us: 'Don't you put me in one of those dreadful nursing homes. I'll be very unhappy with you.' But now, even he could see that the current situation was untenable. He needed closer care around the clock. We all felt a little guilty when we brought up the suggestion: 'How about a bit of a respite?' There was a new building at Regis Burnside, the place my mother had been, and the new facility looked really nice. We all hated the idea, after his complaints about 'those dreadful places'. We stewed over it and talked about it and tried to dream up workable alternatives. But the truth was Dad needed far more attention than we could give him, and all of us had very busy lives. Reluctantly, Dad agreed to give the place a try. We drove him over and helped to move him in.

To our surprise, he didn't seem to mind it. He quickly got to know some of the other residents. He bonded instantly with the staff. People thought he was warm and funny and immensely likable – surprisingly down to earth for someone who'd been a prominent local surgeon. I could have told them that. That's who he was, even at this late stage.

I called him as I was packing for Thailand. 'Hi, Dad,' I said when he answered the phone in his room. 'How are you today?'

For the next few minutes we talked about his nurse and the food and other day-to-day stuff. Then I asked if he knew about the boys trapped in a cave in Thailand.

'Of course I do,' he answered quickly.

With his memory problems, I didn't know if he was telling me the truth. But it didn't matter. 'I'm going to go on a bit of an adventure,' I told him. 'I've been invited to help those kids.'

He answered right away, 'Good on you. Well done, Bert.'

I smiled. That was exactly what I wanted to hear. Dad always worried about my cave diving, but he was also very proud of me. Every time I announced a new trip, no matter how he was feeling about it, he'd say those three words – 'Good on you.' In fact, we had a bit of a comedy routine we'd perform for each other before and after any diving trip. This time wasn't any different.

'Maybe it's time to give it up,' Dad said. 'Why don't you give up the cave diving?'

'You know what, Dad? I think you're right. I'm going to give it away,' I responded, just as I had a hundred times before.

Over the phone I couldn't see his eyes light up, but I could hear it in his voice. 'Oh, that's great,' he said, before delivering the punch-line. 'Hang on. Hang on. You're not telling me the truth, are you?'

'Uh, maybe not, Dad.'

We'd done this routine more times than I could say, but I knew I could count on his reaction. From his nursing-home bed, Dad was roaring with laughter again. He was so happy for me.

I had other people around me with opinions too, four of them especially. That would be Fiona and our three children: James, twenty-two; Charlie, twenty; and our daughter, Millie, who had just turned eighteen. The kids seemed happy for me. They knew how much I loved cave diving and how much I loved being a doctor. In Thailand, I might get to do both at once. They thought it would be cool for their dad to play a part in saving the boys stuck in the cave. That said, all three of them had busy lives of their own, and they weren't exactly sitting around all day focused on their father's cave-diving adventures. James, a talented musician, was touring with his hardcore band, Reactions. Charlie was into his downhill skate-boarding. Millie had just finished high school and was in America, working at a YMCA camp in Connecticut and planning to study fashion marketing at university. But around our place, Fiona was the one who had the most say.

Even before we sat down and discussed it, I had a good idea what she thought, partly because of things she had said to me over the past few days and partly because I know Fiona. She's my wife. She's also a doctor. Her reaction was informed by both of those facts.

She too had been paying attention to the news from Thailand and to my calls, texts and emails with Craig, Rick and Ben. She seemed especially focused on Rick's notion that there might be some way to dive the boys out unconscious and that I could play a key role in that.

At first, I dismissed the possibility as highly unlikely. But the subject was clearly on Fiona's mind. 'Essentially,' she said in her calm but direct way, 'you're the doctor there. These boys are your patients. You're the anaesthetist. It's business as usual. It's just that you're in a very strange environment. Usually there's more light and less water, and backup if you need it. There will be none of that inside the cave. But you're still the doctor, and they're still the patients. It's critical-care medicine. Just do as you always do. You're treating them one at a time. "I'm done with him. Bring the next one in."'

Fiona wasn't worried about me dying in the cave. Craig and I had been away on plenty of other cave dives. This cave would have its challenges – narrow openings, poor visibility and whatever else – but she had confidence in our ability to manage those risks. What worried her was the shape I'd be in once we were done.

My wife is a highly intuitive person. She understood, far more clearly than I did, what the real risk was.

She put the question directly, as she tends to: 'So what impact will this have on you – emotionally, professionally, personally – if even one of them dies? What happens then? What will our lives be like if those boys start to die?'

It was impossible to know, of course. But I got her point. I had told her about Rick's warning, that we'd better prepare ourselves for the worst imaginable news.

'It's great you want to help,' Fiona said to me. 'But you may not be able to save those children. You might get blamed, completely unfairly. You might blame yourself. That's a reality you may not be able to control. What will you be feeling then? How do you go back to work knowing you killed one of those children? How will other people feel?'

I could imagine as well as she could how future patients might respond. But Fiona was the first to put it into words: 'I don't want Dr Harris to anaesthetise me. He's the one who killed those boys in Thailand.'

7

Special K

Harry

In the entire history of medicine, as far as I knew, only one person had ever been in the water under anaesthetic and survived. His name was Edgar Pask, and he was filmed doing it. A quiet and unassuming man, Pask was a British doctor and military officer who conducted research for the Royal Air Force's Medical Services branch during World War II. I never met him, though I devoured his work while I was training to be an anaesthetist and he became one of my professional heroes. Pask was involved in remarkable and sometimes dangerous experiments, studying such things as the effects of acute hypothermia on high-altitude paratroopers and the best ways to resuscitate drowning service members. He was a doctor who was willing to stir up a bit of controversy if that's what it took to save lives. Most strikingly, he did not hesitate to put his own life on the line.

Pask and his New Zealand-born mentor, anaesthetist Robert Reynolds Macintosh, were at the RAF's Physiological Laboratory at Farnborough when they were asked to test an inflatable life-jacket design. Mae Wests, the jackets were called. Once filled with air, they resembled nothing so much as a heaving female bosom, a delightful collision of maritime safety and curvy early-Hollywood sex appeal. These Mae Wests were designed to prevent unconscious pilots and other aircrew from drowning, should they parachute into the English Channel after their aircraft faced enemy fire. Quite a few Allied crewmen had been found dead, face down in the water, floating in their old-style life jackets with water in their lungs.

So would the new design keep an unconscious person floating face up in choppy waters? Pask and his research team aimed to find out.

Pask considered recruiting volunteers to play dead in the water, but he didn't feel that was an adequate test. He wasn't convinced that his volunteers would behave exactly like an unconscious person. How could he be sure his subjects weren't consciously or unconsciously righting themselves? So he settled on a bolder course. He would be his own subject and do the experiment properly. He would strap on one of the Mae West jackets, then have himself anaesthetised, intubated and thrown into the wave pool at the lab. Under these conditions, how would the vest perform? Now, Pask would really know – or he would once he woke up, anyway. He ordered the entire experiment be shot on film, so he'd have a reliable record. It was highly unusual for an eminent medical researcher to conduct an experiment like that on himself. But Edgar Pask was never conventional – he was much more of a jump-in-the-deep-end kind of guy.

To be sure he'd remain unconscious, Pask used a piece of anaesthetic equipment called a Bain circuit, an extra-long piece of coaxial tubing, to keep ether flowing to him wherever he happened to be floating in the wave pool. And the experiment succeeded. Everyone was thrilled to see that, even unconscious, Pask remained face up in his new Mae West. After running the experiment on himself several times, he then anaesthetised volunteer airmen and confirmed that the life jackets performed as they were supposed to. From that time onwards, the film of Pask's experiments was shown to Allied aircrews to boost their morale and let them know, in Pask's words, that 'something was being done'.

This wasn't an easy experience for Dr Pask. Several times, he sank to the bottom of the wave pool and sucked in a lot of water despite being intubated. When he came out of the pool, he was rushed to the hospital and remained there long enough to regain his composure and his strength. Sadly, Edgar Pask died unexpectedly in 1966 at the age of fifty-three. He was beloved by many of the world's leading anaesthetists, then and now. Hardly anyone outside of the field has ever heard of him. But to me he was a great inspiration and one of the unsung heroes of World War II. And who knew? He might even become a hero of the Thai cave rescue. He'd been the one to show that anaesthesia and water *can* mix.

None of this meant that Rick's leading questions had convinced me. I wasn't in the least bit confident that sedating the children was even possible two and a half kilometres into a pitch-dark, flooded cave, much less a safe way of diving them out. Would I even be able to see my young patients well enough to jab the needle in the right place? What germs and bacteria were dancing around in all that cave water? A flooded cave is anything but a sanitary environment. Every five minutes, another objection popped into my head.

If I had to do this – and I meant *if* – how would I do it? First of all, what drug would I use to sedate the boys? I considered lorazepam.

Too long-acting. I considered midazolam. Too unpredictable. I considered clonidine. Not potent enough. Then I started thinking about a drug called ketamine.

Ketamine goes by many names. Ketalar is the most common, though the label could just as easily say Ketaminol, Ketanest, Ketaset, Calypsol, Tekam or Vetalar. Whatever the brand, it's all the same stuff. Ketamine has proven itself over the past fifty years as a reliable sedative in the operating theatre. A shot of ketamine, either intravenously or into the muscle, will send a patient into a trancelike state while also providing pain relief and hypnosis. It's a nice drug with relatively few side effects. Blood pressure, breathing and airway reflexes – generally speaking, they all remain pretty stable.

Though new anaesthetic drugs keep appearing and many of them have grabbed their share of the market, ketamine has never really gone away. Synthesised in 1962, ketamine was first tested on human prisoners in 1964 – the year I was born. Following its approval six years later by the US Food and Drug Administration, the drug was used to anaesthetise wounded American soldiers during the Vietnam War. It quickly found a place for itself in the dispensaries of the anaesthetic departments of hospitals around the world. It wasn't the subtlest or most sophisticated drug, but it was safe, predictable and easy to work with. For those same reasons, veterinary surgeons also started using ketamine to sedate horses and other large animals, and eventually added dogs, cats, rabbits, rats and other smaller creatures to the K-list.

I talked with Craig about this. He'd had plenty of experience using ketamine with his four-legged patients. In fact, he'd used more of it in his practice on animals than I ever had in mine on humans. But both of us had the same feelings about the drug. It was a reliable workhorse and relatively difficult to screw up. In a pinch, amateurs might even be able to administer it.

Like many other drugs meant for medical use, ketamine has also found its way onto the street. With names like Special K, Vitamin K, Kitty and kai-jai, it has developed quite a following on the international club scene, where exhausted ravers value it as a way of coming down after a long, frantic night on the dance floor – or so I'm told. Because of its capacity to cause confusion and amnesia, it's also achieved some infamy as a date-rape drug.

But despite ketamine's colourful and occasionally sordid past, I thought it might be just the ticket here, if all the other rescue options proved even worse. Ketamine is fast-acting. The effects typically begin within thirty seconds after IV injection. Ketamine had a couple of other advantages, too, that might be important in an unpredictable environment like a flooded mountain cave with a group of patients who couldn't be thoroughly pre-screened. Ketamine can be given intramuscularly. No need for the added precision of intravenous injections. And ketamine is a very forgiving drug. The dosage doesn't have to be all that exact. I don't recommend trying it at home, but it's more difficult to overdose a patient on ketamine than some other anaesthetics.

Ketamine's major problem for our purpose, as far as I was concerned, was that its effects don't last all that long. After half an hour or so, depending on the dosage, it's common for a patient on ketamine to rouse. This could be a problem for extracting the boys from the cave. There was no way one injection was going to last for the three or more hours I figured it could take to get each of the boys out. Somewhere along the way, they'd most likely need to be given a top-up dose. Maybe once. Maybe several times. Who would do that? How would they do it, and where? I had no idea. But without top-ups, the boys were sure to wake up on the way out of the cave, creating who-knows-what panic and mayhem, and putting everyone in danger, including themselves.

With all this bouncing around in my head, I decided to seek an outside opinion. Sedate these children inside a flooded cave and dive them out somehow? I needed a reality check. Was Rick's idea just crazy? Could it actually work? And what about ketamine? Was that the right drug? Was there something better out there? I contacted a good friend and colleague of mine in Adelaide, country GP James Doube. James is an inventive jack-of-all-trades, a real-life MacGyver who can come up with a solution to almost any challenge laid in front of him. He has a wider variety of skills than anyone else I know – an expert in everything from organic chemistry to engine repair. He'd spent nearly four years in the Antarctic and on Macquarie Island, a Tasmanian ecological reserve about halfway between New Zealand and Antarctica with a human population of twenty to forty people (and more penguins passing through than anyone would dare try to count). He keeps going back – and not just as a doctor. Sometimes, he's down there driving boats or doing pest eradication. He knows plenty about pesticides and insecticides. He also helps scientists collect data on a broad class of carnivorous, fin-footed, semiaquatic marine mammals formally known as pinnipeds. You and I call them seals.

As part of that research, James is sometimes called on to jump on the back of one of the animals and stick a needle into its spine, pulling blood samples from the epidural veins. That's tough enough with the regular-size fur seals, who are rarely much taller than a metre or heavier than forty-five kilograms. But he also jumps on elephant seals, who can grow up to five metres and over 3000 kilograms.

'It's a relatively safe thing to be doing,' he told me one day, 'as long as they don't roll over and crush you.'

Oh. Okay, then. Just don't ask me to help!

James added that sometimes the scientists toss a modified butter-fly net over the elephant seal's head. 'Like a bag,' James said. 'It seems to calm them a little.'

Hmm, I thought to myself. *That's worth remembering.*

I knew that James had occasionally been asked to anaesthetise a seal, and I remembered him telling me about one he'd put under with ketamine while he was working in the Antarctic.

'James,' I said when I got him on the phone, 'I want to run something by you. You've done a lot of weird stuff with anaesthesia in strange places.'

'I guess so.' He couldn't dispute that.

I told him I was heading to Thailand, where I might be called on to anaesthetise some kids stranded in a flooded cave. 'What do you think about the idea of giving them some ketamine before diving them out?'

'Remember that story I told you about the seal who got away, the one that kept swimming even though he was totally out?' he asked.

'How could I forget?' I said.

The seal had escaped and jumped in the water. James was worried that it was going to drown. But no. Though it seemed to be sleeping soundly, it kept swimming around, its nose out of the water, apparently breathing comfortably.

'Even when he was underwater, he was still looking out for his own airway,' James said. 'I think your kids should be fine.'

'That's very reassuring, James,' I said sarcastically, though I did in fact take some comfort in the wacky anecdote.

'They should do at least as well as the seal,' he said.

That, right there, was the closest thing to actual relevant experience, good or bad, that anyone anywhere had been able to share with me, even though it involved a seal and not a child. The story didn't relieve my doubt, not by a long shot. But my old friend's words did inch me towards the view that this notion of Rick's might not be totally absurd.

I had no idea if the children in Thailand would behave like South Pole pinnipeds. But my own personal MacGyver seemed to think they would.

8

Flying High

Harry

We had quite a ride ahead.

My Qantas flight left Adelaide on Thursday at 6.05 p.m. for the quick hop to Melbourne's Tullamarine Airport, where I was going to meet up with Craig for our nine-and-a-half-hour, overnight flight to Bangkok. But as Thai Airways TG 462 started boarding around 10.30 p.m. at Melbourne's Terminal 2, Craig's plane still hadn't arrived from Perth. We'd texted before he'd taken off and I knew his flight had been delayed, but I was still hoping he'd make it to Melbourne in time. The government travel agency had booked us into business class, which was nice of them, and I wanted to use the flight time to strategise with Craig about the high-stakes adventure we had somehow talked our way into.

But as I settled into my roomy aisle seat, still no Craig.

'I'm waiting for my mate,' I told the hostie. 'It's really important that he gets on this plane.'

I'm not sure how, but she already seemed to know about the situation, where Craig and I were going and what was waiting for us there. She said she would do what she could. She excused herself and made some calls, I believe. Then she came back to my seat and said: 'We can wait another five minutes – but I'm sorry, that's all.'

Craig ended up missing the flight by ten minutes. He had to book another flight a couple of hours later, connecting through Sydney. So there'd be no midair strategising. Each of us would make the trip alone. But it turned out I still had a fellow rescuer aboard.

'You know,' the helpful attendant said to me as soon as the cabin door was closed, 'there's another Australian diver on the plane.'

She pointed out a very fit-looking young man, two rows behind me.

A few minutes after take-off, I wandered back and introduced myself. He said his name was Mark Usback. 'I'm with the AFP SRG,' he said softly. 'I'll be supervising our divers.'

No one had to tell me what AFP was, of course – the Australian Federal Police – though I had a sense there was more to this guy than met the eye. SRG . . . that could mean so many different things, all of them sounding official and slightly mysterious. I found out later it was Specialist Response Group. And Mark had a certain look in his eyes. He was a friendly bloke, but I got the distinct impression that friendly wasn't the only way he was trained to confront the world.

He didn't seem entirely clear – or chose not to say – exactly what their role in the rescue might be. But it was encouraging to connect with such an impressive and seemingly capable bloke. After we'd chatted and I'd returned to my seat, the attendant came round again, this time offering a glass of champagne.

'Well, thank you very much,' I said as I set the glass on my armrest. I retrieved some papers from my bag and, for the first time, began reading my deployment orders, taking the occasional sip of my champagne. I quickly learned there was a huge amount of bureaucratic verbiage required to get two blokes from Australia to help rescue some kids. There were tasking requests and reimbursement policies and the official organisational chart. All the jargon quickly made my head hurt. As I scanned the pages, I accepted the attendant's offer of a refill.

Yes, business class is nicer than economy.

As I was getting comfortable, I couldn't help but notice that AFP SRG Mark was sipping on sparkling water instead of champagne. And maybe this part was my imagination, but he also seemed to be doing a double-take as he looked at me. But we had a long flight ahead of us. So when the attendant offered me another refill, I naturally said yes, as I continued ploughing my way through the government paperwork.

With each sip of bubbly, the bureaucratese seemed even more impenetrable. It was only after I'd caught another one of Mark's glances that I came across the first reference to the Australian government's code of conduct.

Uh-oh! Why hadn't anyone mentioned that?

What it said precisely was: 'The deployed officer, Dr Richard Harris, will be made an employee of the Australian government for the duration of the deployment and will be required to abide by the Australian government code of conduct.'

And also: 'This is a dry mission. Consumption of alcohol is strictly prohibited.'

Really? A dry mission? And I was just learning this after my third glass of champagne?

Ah, now Mark's sideward glances made a lot more sense to me. No wonder he was eyeing me suspiciously. He was probably thinking: *He's got to be an alcoholic. Arrogant prick! Those doctors don't give a shit for the rules.*

I had only two other thoughts before I turned off the reading light and tried to catch some sleep: *No one ever told me this was a dry mission.* And, *Maybe I'll have one more champagne before I drift off.*

Once we landed in Bangkok, I had to ride a shuttle bus from the international to the domestic terminal, where I would pick up my ninety-minute, early-morning Bangkok Airways flight to the regional capital of Chiang Rai. Also on the bus was a strikingly attractive young dark-haired woman who seemed – I swear – to be giving me the once-over, smiling and nodding and acting like she was gathering the courage to speak to me.

My male vanity supplied an answer: *She obviously recognises what a good-looking rooster I am.* I'd momentarily allowed myself to forget that I am in fact a paunchy middle-aged man.

'Are you rescuing the boys or covering the rescue?' she asked, without even introducing herself.

She couldn't have seen what was written on the back of my light-blue button-down shirt: AUSTRALIAN DOCTOR. Or maybe she had, and that's why I'd caught her eye. We were both heading to a place that isn't a huge tourist destination.

'We're *hoping* we can help rescue them,' I said. After Rick's chilling warning, I'd promised myself: no overconfidence. No false optimism. I hadn't even arrived yet. I was in no position to guarantee anything.

The young woman must have picked up on my tone. 'You never know,' she said cheerily. 'It could happen.'

I just nodded at that.

I had my Australian passport in the pocket of my jacket. But since my trip had been thrown together in such a rush, I'd arrived in

Bangkok without a visa or any other official travel documents, other than the stack of stuff I'd got from DFAT. I knew little about my destination and nothing about my accommodation or how long I'd be staying. Should I tick *work* or *vacation* on the entry form? I wasn't sure which. I just hoped that once I'd explained the reason for my visit, some immigration officer would take pity on me. The Qantas agents in Adelaide had looked the other way when I dumped my massively heavy load of excess baggage at the check-in counter – though one of them did sniff sarcastically: 'How many divers do they need over there?' She must have just checked in Mark Usback and all his gear.

My lingering anxiety had eased a bit on the previous leg of the journey. After I got through Sydney Airport's security gate, a young Thai man had come over and introduced himself. He was Kittanu Supasamsen – 'Nu for short,' he said in perfect, polite English. He was a liaison and interpreter working in Thailand for the Australian government. He too was heading to Chiang Rai and then on to Mae Sai for the cave rescue. Nu said his job usually involved getting rowdy Australians out of jail and quickly out of Thailand, so the cave rescue was a new adventure for him. I told him that looking after my dive partner Craig and me might present its own unique challenges, but we would try not to behave like typical Aussies on a Thai holiday.

It was Kittanu who first told me that a 37-year-old former Thai Navy SEAL had drowned early that Friday morning deep inside the cave when something went tragically wrong. Kittanu didn't know exactly what had happened. But he recognised, as I did, that this was an ominous milestone in the rescue campaign.

'The first fatality at the cave,' he said. 'We can only hope it's the last one.'

When our Bangkok Airways flight was finally ready to board, Kittanu and I walked across the tarmac and climbed the aluminium steps to the plane. As we both found our seats – there was no business class this time – I noticed that the young woman from the shuttle bus was a couple of rows in front of me. A few minutes after take-off, she unfastened her seatbelt and turned to talk to me.

'Have you helped rescue people from a cave before?' she asked, still sounding curious.

'Not live ones,' I said.

I didn't elaborate. It was only after we'd landed and were waiting in the aisle to disembark that she tried to draw me out again.

'Don't you think it might be better just to wait out the rain and send in supplies?'

'I think it's better to try,' I said.

She sounded sceptical. 'Men are really going to dive those boys out?' she asked.

'That's the plan,' I said.

She never asked me for my name or exactly what my role might be in the cave rescue. When I asked what brought her to such an out-of-the-way part of Thailand, she said matter-of-factly that she was a journalist working on an article about the rescue for a Canadian magazine.

A journalist? Writing an article? About the rescue? That possibility had never occurred to me. I thought she and I were just talking. I thought she thought I was cool. Had our back-and-forth really been an interview? I didn't know, and I didn't ask her. I just clammed up in a hurry after that.

*

I stepped off the plane and onto the aerobridge at Chiang Rai's international airport. I could see through the large glass panes that a light rain was falling on the tarmac. I hated all rain until we got those children out of the cave. I also noticed that others were staring out of the windows too.

What are they looking at? I wondered.

When I stopped, I got a clearer view of what was happening in the drizzling rain. Perhaps a hundred men and women, many of them in military uniforms, were standing solemnly in two groups. Then a Buddhist monk in a saffron robe walked between the two groups, followed by eight uniformed men – a Thai military honour guard in grey helmets and fatigues, holding an ornate wooden casket draped with the red, white and blue stripes of Thailand's flag.

It was a send-off ceremony for the dead Navy SEAL. What else could be so solemn and so grand?

The people on the tarmac all stood in silence, as those of us inside stared out at them. The light rain kept falling. Hardly anyone moved. Finally, the honour guard stepped forwards and carried the flag-draped casket towards a Royal Thai Navy plane.

I still didn't know many details about what had happened to the former SEAL. But gazing out at the tarmac, I saw what was at stake in this mission I would soon be taking on.

Not just the lives of a dozen children and their young assistant coach, but the lives of all who were coming together to rescue them, including mine and Craig's.

As I wheeled my heavy load of gear out of baggage claim, Kittanu and I were met by two earnest young Australians named Michael

Costa and Cameron Lindsay. Their business cards said they were economic-policy advisers, but they confided that they were on short-term deployment with DFAT's crisis-response team. Their stern demeanour and ever-present notebooks made me wonder: what was the crisis they were responding to? The stranded children or my arrival in Thailand? With the assistance of Kittanu and the local branch of the AFP, they would be on Craig and me like flies on a turd.

Once the gear was loaded and we'd all climbed into the DFAT van, I announced to Michael, Cameron and Kittanu: 'Okay, take me to the cave. I want to go straight to the cave.'

They quickly made it clear to me that this was not the plan. As we pulled out of the airport and began the one-hour drive north on Route 1 to Mae Sai, Michael and Kittanu explained. Since I had shown up with so little warning, there were still some important documents that had not yet been signed. The most pressing was my authority to practise medicine in Thailand. I was an accredited specialist anaesthetist in Australia, of course, but you can imagine how much weight that carried in Thailand. I would need explicit permission from the Thai government to hand out so much as an aspirin in Mae Sai. The DFAT guys had filled out the paperwork on my behalf, they said. But the final sign-off was in the hands of the Thais.

'Until we hear something,' Michael cautioned, 'it really might be better for you to remain in the hotel.'

Oh, great! I thought. I had finally arrived in Thailand. The boys were still trapped in the cave. No one could say when the skies might open again and drown everyone. And where would I be? I'd be under hotel arrest, strictly forbidden to wander any further than the lobby. What sense did that make?

Sorry, lads! Can't help rescue you yet! But I did just call for fresh towels!

The van took us to the Wang Thong hotel (air conditioning, bar fridge, free wi-fi), which was just outside Mae Sai's teeming market and less than a two-minute walk south of Thailand's busy border with Myanmar. I arrived a little after 4 p.m., our trip slowed by the Friday-afternoon bumper-to-bumper traffic heading both ways. I checked into the hotel, unpacked my luggage and my diving gear and then waited. Thirty minutes passed. Then sixty. I called Michael, asking if he'd heard anything. He hadn't. I called again half an hour later. Soon, he promised. Soon. Around seven-thirty, as it was getting dark, he finally called me.

'We have it,' he said. 'You've been approved.' I wasn't sure exactly what I was approved to do, but I didn't see any advantage in nailing down the details. I'd been sitting in my hotel room for two solid hours, ready to go. Craig would be coming soon, Michael assured me, but I didn't want to wait. I left my gear in the room and climbed into the van with my minders for the fifteen-minute drive to the cave.

'Craig can meet us up there,' I said.

The van turned right off the two-lane highway and onto the bumpy road to the entrance of the cave, but I hardly noticed the landscape. I could take that in later. I kept glancing up at the heavy clouds hanging above. The air was close and muggy. There was no telling when those clouds might open up with another burst of monsoon rains.

As we got closer, cars and TV-satellite trucks were everywhere. It looked we were driving up to a music festival or the AFL grand final. People were walking in twos and threes and larger groups along the small road. There were vendors selling plastic bottles of water.

There were people in army fatigues, soccer jerseys, simple dresses and diving gear. There were women standing over pots of hot food. There were boys kicking a soccer ball – boys about the same age as the ones trapped in the cave. And media people. And more media people. And more media people still. There were people everywhere.

I climbed out of the van and stepped straight into a sea of reporters, producers, presenters and what must have been a dozen TV cameras, all pointing at me.

'How are the boys?'

'What condition are they in?'

'How much longer can they survive in there?'

'Are you going into the cave?'

'What's the best option at this point?'

'How long do you expect the rain to hold off?'

I didn't know the answers to any of those questions. I had nothing to tell the media. They had been at the scene for days, and I had just arrived. What was I supposed to say?

'Michael,' I muttered under my breath, 'just take me straight to where the British divers are. I want to talk to the British divers.'

That's all it took. Michael led me to a squat concrete-block building, surrounded by several others like it. It had, until recently, been a rangers' office for the Tham Luang–Khun Nam Nang Non Forest Park. Now, it was headquarters for the growing contingent of British divers on the scene. Open glass louvres. Concrete floor. Fluorescent lighting. Mismatched plastic chairs. Dirty caving gear piled haphazardly on the floor. And a dank aroma that pervaded it all. Somehow, the Brits had commandeered this compact bunker for themselves. What it lacked in style and comfort, it more than made up in proximity, just up the hill from the muddy entrance to the cave.

'Hey, mate!'

It was the cheerful voice of Rick Stanton, greeting me like the old friends we were. He couldn't have been more welcoming, asking about my flight from Australia, Craig's missed connection and what had taken me so long getting out of the hotel.

At Rick's side was John Volanthen. An IT guy who grew up in Brighton and works in Bristol, John is an ultramarathon runner with a dry sense of humour and excellent technical skills. Quiet but opinionated, he's been diving since he was a scrawny Scout. In 1990, he and Rick, along with Jason Mallinson and René Houben, set a world record for the longest distance into a cave, 8800 metres in Spain's Pozo Azul. In 2004, the two of them set a record for the deepest dive in a British cave, 76 metres at Wookey Hole in Somerset, then surpassed this to reach 90 metres the following year. Rick and John both took part in the (unsuccessful) attempt to rescue Éric Establie from the Dragonnière Gaud cave in south-eastern France in 2010, and the successful recovery of the body of Polish cave diver Artur Kozłowski in Kiltartan, Ireland, in 2011.

I was honoured to meet JV, as Rick always referred to John. His is one of the names you just know from moving in these circles – really one of the legends. We'd exchanged emails over the years, especially about an ingenious homemade mapping device he'd invented, but we'd never actually met. He seemed pleased to meet me and excited that he'd soon be meeting Craig as well.

'You heard about the Navy SEAL?' Rick asked me.

I told him I had.

He said he and John had met Saman Gunan soon after they'd arrived at the cave. 'He was a lot like so many of these volunteers,' Rick said. 'Just a tremendous amount of heart, ready to jump in and help, even at risk to themselves. It's hard not to take his death personally. It makes everything seem more real to the rest of us.'

With Michael from DFAT in tow, John gave me a quick tour of the area, trying to steer clear of the media. They showed me where the Australian Federal Police tent was, and I ducked inside. That's where I was, introducing myself to the AFP divers, when Craig appeared.

'Oh, you finally made it,' he said, as if he weren't the one who'd missed his connecting flight and landed in Thailand hours after I did.

'G'day, dickhead,' I said in kind.

Craig had arrived straight from the airport. No hotel arrest for him. All his gear was still in the van he came in. When the driver told him I was at the cave site, that's where he immediately asked to go. It was almost 9 p.m. by then.

'What have I missed?' Craig asked. He doesn't like missing things.

'Nothing, mate,' I answered. 'Just getting started.'

9

Hi, Mum

Harry

As soon as Craig and I trudged up the hill to the British bunker, Chris Jewell and Jason Mallinson came staggering in, just back from a food-delivery run. They were dripping in their wetsuits, still carrying their cylinders, their fins and their masks, looking thoroughly knackered from the long dive they had taken and the short hike up the hill.

Chris and Jason were two of the most experienced and highly skilled members of Britain's long-running Cave Diving Group, deeply driven underwater explorers who'd dived with Rick and John for years. Chris, a 35-year-old computer-software consultant from Cheddar, Somerset, had already been an avid caver before he turned to cave diving in 2006 and started organising diving expeditions into deep, vertical caves. Jason, an amazingly fit 50-year-old dad of a toddler, was a dour Yorkshireman from Huddersfield whose day job as a rope access technician involved hanging off the sides of large structures and required many of the same skills needed in climbing and caving. He had helped Rick rescue six

British soldiers from Mexico's Cueva de Alpazat cave system back in 2004. In 2013, Jason had returned to Mexico with Chris and spent seven weeks in the southern state of Oaxaca, exploring the Huautla cave system in the Sierra Mazateca mountains with a large group of other cavers and divers. The team had towed their camping equipment through a 600-metre underwater tunnel, then assembled their diving gear on a rickety platform above a swirling pool. They slept underground for ten days at a time and made a series of deep decompression dives. But all their efforts paid off when the team established Huautla as the deepest cave in the Western Hemisphere. Now, in Thailand, they found themselves diving in an even brighter spotlight.

'We got some rations from the US Air Force guys, a bunch of high-protein, high-sugar, high-energy stuff,' Chris said. 'First, we separated the rations from the padding around them and the packaging they were in, et cetera. Then, we found our own dry-tubes and crammed the US rations into them.'

'The kids were very happy to see us,' Jason added. 'Better make that *happy to see the food*.'

The boys had been eating far more than anyone had expected. 'We thought we had them supplied for one to two weeks,' Rick said. 'They went through that food in four days. There's been a bit of diarrhoea and some upset stomachs, but nothing too severe – not yet, anyway. They're just hungry, I guess.'

All this was important, I knew. Though they'd been drinking the water that was slowly flowing past their feet, the kids had been without solid food for the first ten days. They needed food for energy. Their bodies craved nutrition. I wasn't an expert, but I knew they were at risk of something that the medical books call *refeeding syndrome*. Starving people who are fed too much too soon can suffer dizziness, seizures, coma and even heart failure. The boys had been fed now, so what was going to happen was going to happen, but we'd need to watch them carefully. Refeeding syndrome can be fatal, but it may take a few days for the signs to appear. However long it took to get them out of there – and no one had a clue yet how long that might be – it was crucial the kids remain as healthy as they possibly could. Rescuing them would be far more difficult and far more dangerous if they started falling ill.

The biggest news that day, though, was that Chris and Jason had notes from the boys and Coach Ekk to pass on to their families. It hadn't been planned, Jason explained – it had been completely impromptu. One of the Thai Navy SEALs had given him a pen and a pad of wet-notes – a special kind of waterproof paper – so he could make notes about the state of the kids' health. While they were in the cave, he'd thought, *You know what? It might be good to have them write something to their parents.* So he told them, 'Here you go. Half a page for each of you. Write a message to your mum or dad or whoever you want to, anything you want to say. Just put it on the pad. We'll take it out with us and give it to them.'

Each of the boys got busy scribbling away on the specially treated paper, trying to ease their parents' concerns in two or three well-chosen lines.

Mum and Dad, I love you, please don't worry. I am safe now. Love you all. – Pong
Mum and Dad, don't worry about me, please, I am fine. Please tell Pee Yod, get ready to take me to eat fried chicken. – Titan
Mum and Dad, I love you, and I love Nong too. If I can get out, please take me to eat crispy pork. Love you Mum, Dad, Nong. – Nick

The boys all signed with their nicknames. Each of them had one, as many Thais do. The sentiments they expressed were so childlike, so simple, so pure, it was possible to read their words and to feel ever so slightly like you knew them. As far as the public was concerned – as far as the *rescuers* were concerned – these little notes were our first real introduction to the boys. Not as team members. Not as Wild Boars. Not as the 'those poor Thai boys trapped in the flooded cave'. But as individuals. From the start, that had been one of the peculiarities of the drama at Tham Luang. The story was so gripping, so human, so easy to relate to – and yet no one outside of Mae Sai really knew these boys as anything beyond 'the boys'.

These little notes provided an early glimpse, and everyone devoured them.

Please don't worry, Mum and Dad. I have been gone for two weeks. I will come back and help you with the shop when I can. I will try to come soon. – Biw

I love you, Mum and Dad, please don't worry about me. I love you all. – Night

Mum, are you well at home? I am fine. Please tell my teacher as well. Love you, Mum Nam Hom. – Mark

Mum, Dad, Brother and Sister and family, please don't worry, I am very happy. – Tee

I am fine, it is a bit cold, but don't worry. Please don't forget my birthday. – Dom

No need to worry about us any more. I miss you all. I really want to go out so much. – Adul

Don't worry. I miss you all, Grandpa, Aunty, Dad, Mum and Nong. I love you all. I am happy, the SEAL team is taking care of us very well. Love you all. – Mix

I love you, Mum and Dad, please don't worry. I can take care of myself. – Tern

I am safe, please don't worry. I love you, Mum, Dad and everyone. – Note

Coach Ekk wrote two notes, the first to his aunt and grandmother:

Dear Aunty and Grandmother, I am fine, please don't worry about me too much. Please take care of your health. Please tell Grandmother to make crispy pork skin with dipping sauce for me. I will come and eat it when I get out. Love you all.

In his second note, Coach Ekk reflected on just how deeply he took his responsibility for the boys:

Dear parents, we are all fine. The team is taking care of us very well. I promise that I will take the best care of the boys. Thanks for all your support and I apologise to all the parents.

Who could read a note like that and not feel torn for this obviously caring young man?

As happy as the notes would certainly make the families, there was a darker possibility here, as well. It struck Jason as he was collecting the papers from the boys. What if they were stuck in the cave for weeks or months or longer? What if they never came home again? As everyone knew, we were only one rainstorm away from true catastrophe. Given the boys' uncertain futures, these short, hastily scribbled messages truly might be the families' final connection with their lost sons.

It was a huge responsibility for all concerned.

This was no argument against having the children write to their families, no argument against diving the short letters out. It wasn't even an argument against the parents sharing the notes with the media, as they did almost immediately. But it was hard not to think about all these possibilities as Jason and Chris relaxed with their mates back in the British bunker while the SEALs, the coach and the children remained behind in the cave.

I was happy to hear Chris and Jason's vivid report, happier still for the families who'd finally had some personal contact with the children they hadn't seen for two weeks now. To be honest, though, I was more interested in talking with Rick and his guys about how we were going to get the kids out of the cave. Of course they needed food and water, and writing notes to their families would keep their spirits up, but the most important thing was getting them out of there as soon as possible. 'Okay,' I said to Rick. It was nearly midnight by then. 'Can we sit down and talk this through? Where are we up to? What's the plan?'

The concrete bunker wasn't much of a conference room, but we pulled some plastic chairs into a circle and got right to it. Besides Craig and I, there were Rick and John, Chris and Jason, plus Derek Anderson and Charles Hodges from the US Air Force Pararescue service – the PJs they called themselves, for parajumpers. The Americans had rushed to the scene and, while they weren't doing much diving, they had quickly proven themselves expert coordinators and organisers, providing a much-needed measure of order amid the chaos outside the cave. They were natural leaders. At one point, British cavers Gary Mitchell and Vern Unsworth popped in. Michael Costa, our DFAT minder, was in the room with his notebook, scribbling down everything that was said.

Rick spoke first. 'Okay,' he said. 'A quick update on where things stand.'

He breezed through all the stuff we already knew. That after the divers had spent several days laying guide rope and searching for signs of life, he and John had located the boys on Monday. That they were stranded on a muddy shelf, just past a stretch of the cave known as Pattaya Beach, which was usually dry but had flooded after the rains. That all the boys were alive and seemed fairly healthy, mentally and physically. That a four-man Thai Navy SEAL team, including a doctor, had been looking after them since Tuesday. That food and other supplies were being ferried in. 'We're stocking up the larder as full as we can,' Rick said, 'not knowing how much longer they're going to be there. And of course, everyone is hoping it won't rain again.'

At Tham Luang cave, the subject of the rain hung over everything. Rick's tone suggested that whatever else was said, all bets would be off as soon as the skies opened again.

'Anyway,' he continued, 'we've been putting together a plan, a detailed recipe for how we think we can get the kids out. I believe you guys know about some of this,' he said, looking at Craig and me. 'Some of it maybe not. If you're ready, we can run you through it now.'

'Eager to hear it,' Craig said.

Rick jumped right in. 'The plan revolves around you getting to the kids and sedating them for the dive out,' he said. 'If you can do that, our guys will dive them out.'

'Before they regain consciousness,' John added.

'*Before*,' Rick agreed.

Rick's plan was to outfit each of the boys in full diving gear. Air tank. Full face mask. Wetsuit. A harness and buoyancy-compensation device to keep them floating horizontally. The divers had clearly worked through many of the details already. I could tell that.

'Positive-pressure full face masks,' Rick said, 'so they can breathe as normally as possible. And front-mounted cylinders.'

'Okay,' I responded tentatively.

He moved on to the next part of the plan. 'Two divers per kid,' he said. 'One in front. One behind. We figure the trip should take a couple of hours. We'll dive them out as quickly as we can. We can probably do six of them the first day. Bang, bang, bang, one after another, moving swiftly through the cave. We don't want anyone waking up before we get them out of there.'

'Wait a second,' I said. 'Two divers per kid?'

I had concerns about that. To me, it sounded like a traffic jam.

'We haven't seen the cave ourselves,' I began, 'so I can't be sure whether what we are sensing is right or wrong. But to me, it sounds like a very dangerous way to do it. There are all these choke points and restrictions in there, right? What happens when one of the kids starts to wake up or panic or flail around? You're going to stop and try to fix that problem. You have a diver in the front, a diver behind. You're in zero visibility. You're not going to be able to see each other. You won't be able to communicate. And then the next bunch of guys are going to bump into you from behind, and then the next bunch of guys are going to bump into them from behind. Before you know it, I can see three dead kids and some dead divers. No one will have any idea what's happening. No one will know what to do. Communication will be impossible. It just sounds like a very dangerous, overly complex way to do it – a potential clusterfuck, as I see it.'

Well, that was met with quiet stares.

It's always dicey raising objections to someone else's plan. Craig and I had just arrived in Thailand. We were the new guys at the cave. Rick and his team had been there for days, working diligently, making progress, winning converts, proving themselves. They knew the cave. They had found the children. And oh, by the way – they were also the most talented and highly respected cave divers in the world. Craig agreed with all of that. Now Craig and I were coming in and pissing all over their carefully crafted plan. But I didn't feel like I had a choice. If we were going to be involved in the rescue, especially if we were being asked to do something so dangerous and completely unprecedented, I couldn't sit there quietly, nodding dumbly along. There could easily have been some pushback against the criticisms I had offered. I would have understood. But that wasn't how they reacted at all.

Rick was still gazing at me intently, but he didn't seem resentful. I knew he'd listened to every word I said and was considering the points I'd made. He wasn't agreeing. He wasn't disagreeing. He just nodded deliberately, as if to say, *Go on.*

So I did.

'I'd like you to consider the possibility of one diver and one child,' I said. 'And a good amount of separation between them. I wouldn't try to do too many in a single day.'

'One diver?' Jason interrupted. He sounded sceptical.

'One diver is better than two,' I said.

That was a lesson Craig and I had learned the hard way seven years earlier, diving our good friend Agnes's body out of Tank Cave, when I ended up in an alcove with Craig behind me pushing forwards. It was a frightening lesson we'd never forget. That dive was much shorter than this one would be. And sadly, of course, we didn't have to worry about Agnes's breathing, or whether water was seeping into her mask.

'You're trying to do something complicated,' I said. 'But you can't communicate when something starts to go wrong. You can't even see each other well enough to trade hand signals. You can't say, "Stop and wait while I fix this." You can't tell if the guy in front of you is all right, and he can't tell if you're all right.'

All of that had been a challenge for Craig and me with Agnes. The problems would be multiplied here.

'Say you're at the back,' I said. 'You'll feel the child thrashing around. You can tell something's going wrong. But you can't see or feel exactly what the problem is. Is it that I can't get through the opening in front of us? Is it that I'm worried about the kid and I've turned around? Have I lost the line? Are we now off the line, and I'm the bloke who's supposed to be navigating? Are we lost now? Any number of things could be going wrong. If you can't even see each other to work out how to solve that problem right away, things are going to disintegrate. You're trying to do what you think is the right thing to fix the problem. I'm trying to do what I think is the right thing to fix the problem. I'm worried about you, but I don't know what's happening to you. You're a metre out of my reach, no more than the length of a child's body, but we might as well be a mile apart from each other. I've got a kid who's starting to wake up or might be panicking. I don't know if you're there or not. It could be anything. Everything can go pear-shaped really, really fast.

'It all gets easier,' I said, 'when it's one on one. If it's just me and the kid, I know that I'm the one who has to keep hold of that line or I'm in trouble. I'm not taking my mind off anything, assuming that you'll keep an eye on it – not even for a second. If the kid starts to have a problem, I can lock the line under my arm and try to sort it out. If I come to a pinch point that requires a bit of feeling around to work out exactly how to get through, I can take as long as I need to without worrying about the guy behind me, who I know will be worrying about what's happening up front with me. And in the worst-case scenario . . .' – I hated to even raise the possibility, but how could I not? – 'if the kid drowns, I'll deal with that and keep moving forwards. Once you're in the water with the boy, that's what you're going to have to do. There will be no turning back.'

I knew I had given quite a speech there. I really didn't mean to land in Thailand and lecture everyone. But this was no time to put a sock in it. I didn't think what I was proposing would seem all that radical, not to world-class cave divers. Much of cave diving is done solo, a far safer way of doing things when the cave is tight, the visibility is bad and you're not sure what you are going to find. Even when you step into the water with a partner, that doesn't mean you'll swim right beside each other throughout the entire dive. Underwater in a cave, a little distance can actually be your friend. It's not like you're carrying on long conversations with each other. Cave diving might be a team sport, but it's fundamentally a solo act. You can watch each other's backs. You can help in an emergency. But if you don't have a second diver right there next to you to worry about, you can slow down and do everything at your own speed. It's easier to focus. It's a lot less complex. Having your mind in a space where everything is simplified is a huge safety benefit.

And apparently, Rick didn't disagree. 'Okay,' he finally said. 'I see what you mean.' He seemed to appreciate that I hadn't just dismissed their plans out of hand. I'd offered what I believed was a practical alternative and carefully laid out my reasoning. I understood that Craig and I weren't there for our diving prowess. Rick and his guys were unmatchable. We were there primarily because of our medical expertise. But our insights were an added bonus, I suppose, and the Brits were still willing to listen to us.

There was some discussion of my one-diver-one-boy proposal, but less than I would have expected. Soon, everyone was saying, 'Okay, that sounds all right.'

Not bad for our initial meeting. No major blues or anything. Now all we had to settle was everything else.

10

Question Everything

Harry

The British didn't get to decide. The Americans didn't get to decide. Craig and I didn't get to decide. Coach Ekk and the boys definitely didn't get to decide. Any rescue plan, whatever it was, would need the explicit approval and support of the Thai government. The Thai medical authorities. The Thai foreign ministry. The Thai first responders. And most of all, it seemed, the Thai military. We weren't in charge. They were.

Craig and I had both been to Thailand several times before. It is a beautiful country with an ancient culture and some of the gentlest and most welcoming people on earth. From the 24-hour mega-capital of Bangkok to the world-class beach resorts of Phuket to the temples and shrines of the north, Thailand is an intensely spiritual and thoroughly global country where the traditional and the modern live side by side every day.

The Kingdom of Thailand, as the nation is officially called, is a constitutional monarchy, which is why many of its institutions, including the Royal Thai Army, the Royal Thai Navy and the

Royal Thai police, still have the word *royal* in their names. Though the kings and queens were stripped of their power in the revolution of 1932, the monarchy was not abolished, and they are still revered figures in Thailand. Since that time, real power has resided in a succession of military leaders installed after coups d'état, the most recent in May 2014, with a few democratic intervals along the way.

As the Tham Luang drama began, Thailand was ruled by a military junta, the National Council for Peace and Order. The Thai military authorities at first were confident that their own military and first responders could handle everything. But the generals quickly came to recognise, especially after Saman Gunan died, that a flooded cave was a uniquely perilous environment that Thai personnel didn't have the training to handle alone. This was a job that called for high-level international expertise and cooperation, though the Thais would never give up ultimate control.

In navigating all this, we did have one secret weapon: Josh Morris.

An American from Utah who ran a caving and climbing business in Thailand, Josh was married to a well-connected Thai woman and spoke fluent Thai. He explained to the Thai generals how the international cave divers could be helpful and explained Thai customs and etiquette to the divers. 'There's a Thai word that means "connector",' he said to us. '*Cheǔxm*. It's the same word you use for welding. You need a connector here.'

And with Josh we had one.

Chiang Rai governor Narongsak Osottanakorn was put in charge of the overall rescue at an operational level. Though he'd recently been ordered to wrap up his job as governor of the northern province, he remained on duty to coordinate at the scene. Numerous top

Thai officials, including Prime Minister Prayut Chan-o-cha, a former general, were involved in many of the major decisions. Certainly they had to sign off on any rescue plan.

That was front of mind for Rick and all the rest of us. Whatever we settled on would need the blessing of the military leaders. Otherwise, it wasn't happening. At our first meeting in the British bunker, sedation had definitely been the top contender, but we hadn't settled on anything.

Craig remained a leading sceptic. He wasn't at all convinced that sedation would be necessary. It was still worth exploring, he said, whether the boys could be outfitted in wetsuits and full underwater-breathing gear and dived out of the cave the normal way, each escorted by an experienced diver.

'These kids are tough,' Craig argued. 'Look at how well they've done in the cave so far.'

He had a point. According to the Brits, the boys had been unbe-lievably resilient, maintaining their health, their sanity and their good spirits for two severely challenging weeks. Their team spirit, the guidance of Coach Ekk, whatever it was – under impossible circum-stances, they had held up remarkably well.

'Maybe we should just give it a go,' Craig suggested. 'See how they do in the water. Take them out for a dive. Who knows? They might surprise us all.'

That was pure Craig, putting his faith in the power of human ingenuity and drive. He knew that motivated people, including children, could accomplish amazing things. But could the desire to get out of the cave really carry these boys that far? Cave diving is an inherently risky activity. The consequences of failure are severe. No one else seemed eager to test-drive Craig's let's-just-try-it approach. Even he didn't push the idea too hard. With divers as young and as thoroughly inexperienced as these, he conceded, panic is awfully hard to hold back. A couple of unexpected gulps of water really could change everything.

Craig ended up at the same place as the rest of us. Full sedation, anaesthesia in fact. Positive-pressure face masks. Hands and feet bound. One diver, one boy. Thirteen neat little packages gliding underwater through the cave.

'They'll be experiencing something they've never experienced before,' he admitted. 'It will seem very threatening.'

We hadn't been in the cave yet, but we both knew what to expect. The jutting rocks. The low ceilings. The constricted corners. The narrow openings. We were used to these conditions and would be completely comfortable, but not so the boys.

'Whether they're conscious or not, they'll be banging against rock as they move through the cave. It's inevitable,' Craig said. 'And being unable to see can be pretty disorienting.'

Though the knocks and scrapes wouldn't be life-threatening, they might be painful, and startling enough to shatter a newbie's confidence. Could youthful exuberance or Buddhist calm really stand up to that?

'You can imagine someone coping with it for a short while,' Craig said finally. 'But for hours? That's unrealistic, I suppose.'

I had a couple of small but important suggestions still to add. One thing we should do, I said, was give each of the boys an anti-anxiety medication before the dive, something like alprazolam. It wouldn't knock out the pre-trip jitters entirely, but it would take the edge off them. I'd also give each of them a shot of atropine, which would dry out their mouths, to prevent them choking on their saliva.

Everyone seemed to think both those suggestions were sensible.

Step by step, we were getting closer to a working plan. Now, all we had to do was pull it apart, tweak it, test it and sell it to the Thais.

So was there a middle ground here? That was one question. Did the children have to be *totally* knocked out before they could be dived out of the cave? That was another. Questions. So many questions. They kept coming as the night wore on.

Would light sedation be enough? If so, the boys might still be able to follow simple instructions in the water, control their own breathing and be more attuned to what was happening around them.

Turn right. Go slow here. Okay, now we have to get out of the water and walk across this sandy stretch.

With a little practice, couldn't we teach a slightly medicated boy how to wiggle through a narrow constriction, or to blow water out of his leaky mask?

But the instant that something went wrong – and we all knew that *something* would go wrong – would that mild sedation be enough to stop a child panicking? No, it probably wouldn't, everyone agreed, not if he thought he was about to drown.

Rick reminded us then of what had happened the day after he and John first arrived, when they'd gone into the cave looking for the boys and come upon the four Thai water workers trapped in chamber 3. 'They were absolutely terrified when we tried to dive them out,' he said. 'They were certain they were going to die.'

To escape, the men had to dive through the short sump connecting chambers 3 and 2. It was only ten metres, but the men had no previous scuba experience and Rick and John had to ram them through a half-hour beginner's diving course. It hadn't done much good. The men were too scared to stay and too scared to go. When they'd finally agreed to press ahead, at least two of the Thai water workers had panicked severely, so much so that Rick and John both thought someone might die.

'These were grown men, not children, experienced adults all of them,' John said. 'And they were in chamber three, close to the entrance of the cave. The dive was only about twenty or thirty seconds. Yet they were convinced they wouldn't make it out alive.'

Once they'd stepped out of the cave, all four of the Thai water workers disappeared into the darkness, and neither Rick nor John had seen them since. If this was how four adults reacted, how would a dozen children and their young coach respond?

Hearing that story seemed to strike a chord with most of the people in the room. Each of us had extensive scuba experience, but I'm sure many of us remembered our first cave dives, how strange, difficult or exhilarating they had been. The story was a reminder that we had all spent years in and around the water, and that we'd chosen to be here – none of which could be said for Coach Ekk and his soccer players.

'The reality can't be ignored,' Rick said. 'As long as those children are awake and alert, there's no way they are coming out of that cave without being terrified.'

Under these circumstances, terror meant panic, and panic could be fatal – for the children and even for the rescuers who had come all this way to save them.

After we'd talked things over a while longer, Rick moved in to close the deal. 'So, Harry,' he asked, 'can you do this or not?'

I didn't think Rick was trying to pressure me. Time was ticking by, and he just wanted an answer – *soon*. I was inching closer to one, thoroughly convinced we had to do something without delay. We couldn't just leave those boys in the cave, waiting for the rainy season to be over and the water to subside. No one had any idea how long that might take. All kinds of things could happen between now and then. The boys could get sick. They could become malnourished. They could go crazy. There was no end to the catastrophes that might befall them. The close-as-brothers team members could turn on each other, hard as that was to imagine now. We couldn't wait around for a Wild Boars' version of *Lord of the Flies*. And the monsoon rains could roar in at any minute, making all this rescue talk moot. As for the other ideas that were still kicking around, none of them held much promise any more. The drillers and the drainers had already tried and failed. Somehow or other, cave divers would have to go in there and haul those boys out.

I was on board with all of that.

I was getting more comfortable with the idea of anaesthesia, too. Though I'd been highly sceptical when Rick first ran that idea past me in Adelaide, I had reluctantly come most of the way around. On a long list of terrible options, it really was the best we had. I felt sure that ketamine was the most appropriate drug of all the choices available to me. I felt good about the one-diver-one-boy strategy. I felt good about the skill and professionalism of the divers on Rick's team. We had the best anywhere.

So what was the problem? Who or what was I doubting?

'I can't agree to anything,' I said to Rick and the others, 'until I dive the cave. I need to feel confident I can do it, that I can physically do it. That I'll be in the condition I need to be to do my job. I have to see the place where I'm going to sedate these boys. And I want to meet them. I *need* to meet them.'

'You need to *meet* them?' Jason asked, as if he hadn't quite heard me.

'They'll be my patients,' I said. 'I need to meet them.'

Some of my concerns were medical. Some were psychological. Some were physical.

The truth was I had doubts about my own physical fitness and my ability to operate in the cave. I was pathetically out of shape. I'd put on some extra kilos. I had been ignoring the nagging pleas of Fiona and my children to get my lazy butt to the gym. I had good excuses. I'd been busy at work, with new managerial duties that kept me at my desk so long every day it couldn't possibly be healthy. But the fact remained I hadn't done much diving lately, and it showed. To recognise this, all I had to do was look in the mirror.

'Just look at me,' I said. 'I know you guys are super-fit and lean, and you've been actively caving recently. But I'm a bit out of it. I haven't done a big dive like this for a while. I just need to dive the cave and make sure I can handle everything.'

It was important, I thought, to see exactly where the boys were. Other people had described it to me: the boys and their coach were all crowded together on a ledge up a muddy slope from flooded Pattaya Beach. I could point to it on Vern's map. I could more or less picture it in my head. But none of that was a substitute for diving there and seeing it with my own eyes.

This wasn't just curiosity, though I was curious. Somewhere on the ledge or down below it, I was going to have to set up a make-shift operating theatre where I could anaesthetise each of the boys and prepare them for the unconscious dive out. It would be dark in there. The conditions would be far from sanitary. I wasn't sure if I would have a stable, level place to do the injections. How would I hold the boys and stop them falling prematurely into the water after they were asleep? Was there something I could sit on? Was there a dry spot near the water – dry enough to perform my injections but close enough to the water that the dive could begin right away?

Was there a place where we could lay the boy down while his hands and feet were bound together and other last-minute preparations were made? It was impossible to answer any of these questions without going there.

'You guys have all been in the cave and seen the kids,' I said. 'I think Craig and I should dive the cave tomorrow.'

I got pushback on that, especially from Jason.

It turned out that the British divers had other plans for Saturday – important plans – and wanted Craig and me to come along. They had arranged a rehearsal dive in an indoor swimming pool at a school in Mae Sai about a twenty-minute drive from the cave. As closely as possible, they wanted to duplicate the conditions of the rescue, right down to recruiting three teenagers from a local swimming club to play the roles of the sedated Wild Boars – a small boy, a medium-size boy and a larger one. The Thai Navy SEALs were sending people to watch the rehearsal. So was the US military. Two local paramedic crews had agreed to come with their ambulances, just in case anything went wrong. Various other Thai government representatives, local civic leaders and medical personnel had also promised to attend.

It wasn't quite an Edgar Pask experiment, but it still sounded to me like an excellent idea.

The Brits and Derek Anderson from the US Air Force Pararescue team had clearly thought this out with exquisite precision, right down to the minutest detail. The young volunteers would be dressed in wetsuits and buoyancy vests, just as the Wild Boars would be for the actual rescue. Each boy would have a cylinder full of oxygen strapped to his front and held in place with a modified harness that had a handle on the back – all the better for his escort diver to control the unconscious boy. A lead weight in the front pocket of the harness would keep the boy face down. That was the idea, anyway.

From their own collection and from other divers at the site, the Brits had gathered a variety of face masks in varying sizes – small, smaller and smallest – which they hoped to fit on the different-sized boys.

The divers would test the masks, test the tanks, test the hoses, test the silicone seals and test anything else they could think of. Rick said he would ask his young test subjects to remain perfectly still in the water, as if they were fast asleep. He said he especially wanted to see how they would breathe inside a full face mask the first time their faces were pressed into the water. 'Will they know instinctively to breathe or not?' Rick asked.

MacGyver's seal had. Would the boys?

'That all sounds brilliant,' Craig said to Rick and Jason after they had laid it out for us. The swimming-pool dress rehearsal was a smart idea. It could very well teach us all some lessons – *this* works, *this* doesn't – that would prove lifesaving later on.

'I'll be eager to hear the results of the experiment,' I said.

Jason saw his opening there. 'So come along,' he said. 'Get up in the morning. Take a bit of a dive in the cave. Go halfway in to make sure you feel comfortable with your gear and everything. A standard shakedown. Then meet us at the pool.'

I understood what Jason was saying. It was a good suggestion. But I didn't think I could budge.

If we could somehow have wangled an extra day here, Craig and I would have happily gone back to the pool for a second go-round *after* we had scoped out the inside of the cave. In fact, I had already raised the idea of a full dress rehearsal in a pool, including anaesthesia – no more volunteers *pretending* to be asleep.

Call it a *full Pask*. The ethics of this were sketchy at best, but the Thai military was prepared to sanction it. They even told me they would recruit the 'volunteers' who would be sedated. But all the pressure to get the rescue started and the looming threat of rain made that seem unlikely, if not impossible. We just couldn't risk another day's delay.

'This isn't really negotiable for me,' I said finally to Rick and the others. 'I have to be sure I can dive the cave before I can agree to do anything. I don't know how long the dive is, how well I will do in there. I have to see the state the kids are in. How big or little they are. How healthy or frail. I need to see the exact spot where I'm supposed to anaesthetise them. I have to work out in my own mind whether it's even possible in conditions like these.'

Only then could I agree with a clear conscience that a sedated dive was the only idea left to try.

'You don't want me saying "no way" after we all think everything's a go,' I added.

The Brits finally agreed.

'All right,' Jason said. 'You and Craig do your dive tomorrow. While you're at the cave, we'll have a play-around in the pool.'

On the drive back to the hotel that night, Michael Costa, our diligent DFAT minder, said he had something he needed to mention to us.

'In the interest of full disclosure,' he said somewhat stiffly, 'I have to tell you that if something goes wrong with the children, it's not impossible that you could get caught up in the Thai judicial system.'

'The Thai judicial system?' I repeated slowly, making sure I'd heard him right. 'Like the *Bangkok Hilton*?'

I'm not sure if Michael appreciated my reference to the three-part Australian miniseries, in which Nicole Kidman's character is confined to a hellhole of a prison in the Thai capital. He managed a stiff chuckle, though, and said: 'Well, not exactly.'

The Australian government, Michael explained, had applied to the Thai government for diplomatic immunity for Craig and me while we were working on the rescue. That way, if anything bad should occur, we wouldn't be held legally liable. While our Australian handlers said they had every expectation that our applications would be approved, there'd been no formal word yet from the Thai officials, and no one could say for certain when – or even *if* – the approval might arrive.

This made no sense to me. Hadn't Craig and I *volunteered* to come to Thailand and help these desperate children? We'd be risking our own lives trying to free them from the cave. And we were far from the only ones. There were hundreds of other kind-hearted volunteers – who'd come from almost every country you could name. They were military, civilian, foreign, Thai. With the finest of intentions, they too were here to help.

'What about all these other blokes?' I asked.

'No,' Michael said, shaking his head. 'Mainly you. You're the doctor, and you'll be giving the drugs. So if the children die . . .' He let the thought taper off there, but I was pretty sure I caught his drift. There weren't going to be any thanks-for-trying citations if something unfortunate occurred. There'd be a cosy cell in a Thai prison waiting for me. I had never been incarcerated and didn't really know anyone who had, but with everything else already swirling in my head, I now had the pleasure of imagining what and who might be waiting for me in my cell.

'Are you sure about all this?' I asked Michael.

I was about to go off on him. I had accepted this high-profile mission. I had recruited my good friend Craig. I had put us both on the line. There had never been any guarantee of success. In fact, I wasn't at all sure that something wouldn't go wrong. Swimming sedated children out of a flooded cave was not a foolproof plan. *If the Thais have a better alternative, please, by all means, grab it! I'll bow out and let some other idiot swim in there.*

That was what I was thinking. That wasn't what I said. Instead of erupting like a volcano, I shrugged.

'You know what, Michael?' I said. 'I haven't got the bandwidth to think about this at the moment. I've got too much to think about already. You've got to take care of this. So let's not speak of it again.'

He just stared.

'Seriously,' I said, 'I can't think about this right now. You'll just have to look after me if something goes wrong, right? Scoop me up. Get me out of Thailand. I trust you. I'm in your hands.'

Michael promised he would take care of Craig and me if anything went horribly wrong. At least I think that's what he said. That's the way I heard it, but I had no plans to test his promise anyway, and it was late and I was exhausted, so I didn't ask him to clarify. Craig and I had reached the hotel by then. We were both totally knackered. What a day! We had a dive planned for the morning into a dark and difficult cave.

III

Diving

11

First Dip

Craig

We had studied Vern's map, of course, and a couple of others too. But a map is only the roughest estimation, the vaguest notion of what you'll find inside a cave. Unless you've been there, you haven't been there. No piece of paper, not even a beautifully shot video, can adequately capture the infinite variables inside a cave. The clarity of the water. The hues of the limestone. The sound of the echoes. The heaviness of the air. The size, shape and difficulty of the restrictions. The vital importance of the guide line and the feeling you get when you've dropped it underwater and your heart is pounding and you're trying to keep your composure as you firmly say to yourself: *Everything's fine. I'll retrieve the line in a second. And even if I don't, I'm sure I'll still get out of here.*

I don't care if you're the next Leonardo da Vinci. There is no way to draw that on a map.

Since this was Thailand in early July and we figured the water would be relatively warm, Harry and I climbed into thin surfing wetsuits – *squeezed* into the suit, in Harry's case. (Sorry, mate.)

We had fins, dive harnesses with built-in buoyancy, and various accessories – spare lights, carabiners, extra reels for emergencies – clipped onto D-rings. No full face masks for us, just normal regulators. Each of us carried three side-mounted eleven-litre air cylinders – eighty-eights, we call them – two on one side, one on the other. Three is more than we would normally carry. That slows you down a bit. But this time, we went with the added margin of safety. We wouldn't be able to rescue anyone if we had our own catastrophe inside the cave. This dive had to go well.

Actually, 'this dive' isn't the best way to put it. It wasn't one long dive to the spot where the boys were – it was seven shorter dives, separated by air chambers that we swam or waded through. The tanks alone weighed nearly twenty kilos each – a lot of lugging there. Fortunately a guide line was already in place to lead us in and out of the cave.

Much of the line in this case would actually turn out to be climbing rope. Normally, cave divers use braided string, around 3 millimetres in diameter, to mark their route into the cave, so anyone using it will have a clear path out. But Rick and John had put some line in. Ben did a lot of it as well. They had wisely decided to use the fatter climbing rope, stronger than regular line. They knew that quite a few people would be coming and going from the cave, and not just experienced cave divers. That climbing rope was sure to get an absolute flogging, but it wasn't going to break no matter how many untrained amateurs yanked on it. If they'd used normal braided line, it would have already been in tatters or pulled loose for sure.

Around 11 a.m., Harry and I carried our gear to the entrance of the cave, trying not to attract attention as we wove through the mob of people who were milling around. The crowd had definitely grown in the twenty-something hours since we had arrived.

'Here goes,' Harry said as we made our way into the first chamber of the cave without anyone stopping or even recognising us.

'Let's do it,' I answered.

There isn't much talking on a cave dive. There is none under-water, and not much more at the surface, while you are grunting and struggling into the flowing water. Sporadic cussing is about as sophisticated as the audible communication gets, which leaves hand and light signals, and the occasional tap or nudge, nod or head jerk. This is part of what makes cave diving such a solo sport, even when it's done in teams.

The first half-kilometre was just a hike. Along a stream. Over some rocks and hills. Up steep slopes slick with mud and the drip-pings of other workers and divers. As we secured our masks and stepped into the water, it was just as warm as we had expected – about 23 degrees Celsius. Some of the local divers had said that the water felt cold to them. But given a few of the frigid places Harry and I had gone diving over the years, it didn't feel the least bit chilly to us. We were in a section called a roof sniff, where the water almost reaches the ceiling and you need to haul yourself through with your nose in the air, like a dog swimming, so you can breathe. That's when we reached the first sump. It wasn't long at all, ten quick metres between chambers 2 and 3, but it gave us a clear warning of things to come. We had to slide through a tight flattener – a section in which our backs touched the rock above while our chests were touching the rock below. It was only short, but tight enough that, as Harry and I passed through, you could hear our cylinders clanging against the rock. It's amazing how clearly that sound cuts through water, like an urgently ringing doorbell on an otherwise silent night.

All I could think of as we were banging through was how much harder this would be towing a sedated boy. This was tough for Harry and me alone. It would be a whole lot tougher with an unconscious passenger.

The passage narrowed there, concentrating the myriad water pipes, communications and power cables that had been brought into the cave. It was a chaotic tangle of man-made and natural obstacles. But at the far end of that tight underwater passage was its geological opposite – a huge open chamber.

A steep, gooey mud slope led up to chamber 3, as spacious as a train station, and bustling with activity. It was the inside dive base for the entire rescue mission, a combination warehouse, dormitory, repair shop, relief station and rec hall where divers, technicians, soldiers and assorted support personnel supplied and inventoried damn near everything that went in or out of the cave. A large group of Thai Navy SEALs were living there. They had sleeping-bags. They had plastic bottles of water, and military rations to eat. They had their own communications gear. We didn't see it, but we heard they'd run a fibre-optic internet line in there. And stacked inside chamber 3 were probably 300 dive cylinders. I could hardly believe my eyes when I saw that mountain of tanks. If the circumstances had been different, I'd have sworn I'd just arrived at a Bunnings that could use a little tidying up. I half-expected someone to ask me, 'What aisle are the showerheads in?' For divers like us, heading deeper into the cave, chamber 3 was an oasis.

Though the space was commodious and the ceiling was high, this was exactly where Rick and John had had to rescue the stranded Thai water workers. But our reconnaissance journey had only begun.

'Ready for a nice spot of cave diving?' Harry asked me with a smile.

I nodded that I was, returning the grin. Standard-issue cave-diver sarcasm.

We'd been warned about the next bit of diving in the cave, the section between chamber 3 and chamber 4. This was where Saman Gunan, the former Thai Navy SEAL, had died. Once we reached that spot, it was easy to understand how.

This section was by far the worst part of the cave to dive through – 150 metres long, and extremely difficult to navigate. Rocks projecting from the roof kept cracking against our helmets, even as we tried to anticipate them by waving our hands in front of our faces. There was a T in the line where someone had taken an early wrong turn, up into a tiny air chamber with a blind ending. We had to reverse course and return to the T-junction in order to proceed the correct way. A tricky S-bend through a vertical slit meant we had to slide ourselves through a 3D puzzle that could only be solved by trial and error in the inky blackness of the water. Finally, there was a classic line trap, where the rope had been pulled into a gap so narrow that it was impossible for a diver to follow. We held the rope at arm's length while we groped around in the dark to find a larger hole that would accommodate our girth. Yep, this section was like a cruel obstacle course designed by the most malevolent cave-diving instructor ever!

'Boy, I wouldn't want to be bringing a kid through there,' Harry said after we'd cleared it. 'That was tight for me on my own.'

But we kept moving forwards, partly by swimming, partly by wading. In places, it was easier just to pull yourself along the rope hand-over-hand. That seemed to be the most efficient way to travel. Overall, it would be another kilometre and a half like that. The water was coming at us, with a couple of metres' visibility. Not good and not too bad – for now. On the way out, the visibility would be close to zero, as we'd have stirred up the mud deeper in the cave. Seeing would be a good deal harder, no doubt about it.

There was a spot, about halfway to the boys, that the British divers had told us to look out for. Monk's Junction, it was called on the map. 'It's where the tunnel separates,' Rick said. 'You'll know you're there because all of a sudden, clear, warm water is coming through from the right. You're swimming along through so-so visibility, then the water gets warmer and you can see. It's just for a few metres, but it's noticeable.'

Rick had it exactly right.

Normal temperature, blah visibility, a fork in the tunnel, then – *whoosh!* For a few sweet metres, warm, clear water came rushing in.

As experienced divers, Harry and I knew that meant fresh water was flowing in from a side tributary. The warm, clear water quickly mixed with the muck and faded to nothingness, but it would be a hard-to-miss halfway marker every time we came and went. By comparison, most of the rest of the route, with the exception of chamber 3 and a couple of tight, nasty crawls, was fairly forgettable, no matter how closely we studied the map or how many times we'd pass through. Sump, air chamber, sump, air chamber. But there was no missing Monk's Junction.

Every now and then, we'd trade a sarcastic comment or two.

'Having a good time?' I asked Harry.

'Love the zero viz,' he said.

'We've seen worse,' I reminded him.

'And we may again soon.'

The trepidation was building as we got ever closer to the boys. It was one thing to make plans at a distance for rescuing them. It would be something else to look them in the eye and explain to them exactly what we had in mind. The rescue was getting more real with every rope pull.

After a while, it was hard to know how close we were to our goal. Each time we surfaced into a dry patch or an air chamber, one or the other of us would wonder: *Are we there yet? Are we there yet?* You lose track of how far you've come. We tried to stay alert for certain landmarks. At one spot, we were told, the orange rope would change to flat black tape, and then back to orange rope again. Near the end, there'd be a stretch of thin blue rope. Once we hit the blue rope, we'd know we were close to chamber 9 and the kids.

People had mentioned chamber 4 and chamber 6 and chamber 7. But we'd come up and down, up and down. We didn't know exactly where we were. Some of the sumps were chest-deep, and we waded along on our feet, pulling ourselves along the rope. But half the time, we didn't even know whether there was rock above us, or air, or what we had in front of us at any given time.

Once we reached chambers 7 and 8, we had to climb out of the water and walk again. We kept our tanks on, but the hike was far enough that we took off our masks and fins, carrying the fins in our hands. Gravity sucks when you are carrying gear along a sandy beach and up over rocks.

Again, the thought kept intruding: *How will this be for those who are carrying the boys?*

The last sump we passed through, about 300 metres long, was by far the nicest bit in the cave. This was more like the cave diving we like to do rather than the slog we had just experienced. It was actually quite a pretty dive in that section, a nice refresher before the main event.

Then we reached the thin blue rope.

Rick and John had warned us about the stench in chamber 9.

'As soon as we stuck our heads up,' Rick had said, 'it was putrid in there.'

This made sense. The boys had been in the cave for two weeks by then. Urine. Shit. Sweat. Have you ever been inside a high school locker room? That's what I was expecting to swim into.

As we surfaced, I didn't smell anything. I don't have the greatest sense of smell, though.

'Smells like ammonia,' Harry said. 'Acrid. Is that urine?'

We had emerged into what turned out to be quite a long canal. There was no sign of the boys yet. We kept swimming along the surface with our masks on. Keeping a hand on the rope. Inching ever forward. Finally, on the left, a partly flooded beach came into view. Low. Sandy. Flat. On the right was a ledge. The deep canal dividing them ran on, disappearing into the distance up ahead.

We'd been told there was a beach opposite where the kids were. 'You'll see a hill going up,' John had told us. 'They're up there.' Once we saw the beach, we knew it wouldn't be much longer. By that point, our general unease had risen to genuine anxiety. We had no idea how the boys were going to react to us. What would they say? What would we say to them? How would they respond when we explained the dicey plan we had in mind for them?

'Anything's possible,' Harry said. 'Are they going to panic and attack us and take our gear and swim out with it?' No! We were there to help them. But we'd both read enough books about people trapped on desert islands to know that the best-intentioned rescuers are often tomorrow's lunch. We weren't expecting any live fire in our direction. The Navy SEALs hadn't brought weapons, had they? But still, we approached with extra caution.

We stopped at the beach. We shed the tanks there and pulled off our fins. We knew we had some climbing in front of us. Then we paddled across the water with our masks on. As we glided across the surface, we began to hear voices, just as predicted, off to the right and up ahead. We saw lights. Then we saw people. They were waving. At us.

12

Wild Boars

Harry

'G'day,' I called to the waving boys as I pulled myself out of the water.

'Hello,' Craig said.

'Hi!' the boys called back. It was possible that was all the English most of them knew, aside from a few other stray words.

Now that Craig and I had survived the gruelling two-and-a-half-kilometre dive, there were several pieces of business to attend to. First of all, we needed to observe the stranded boys. I wanted to see with my own eyes whether the children were really as healthy as I kept hearing they were. Was that just wishful thinking? Could it really be true? I didn't expect to perform full medical examinations – that would have been impossible on such a tight deadline, with no medical equipment and in dismal light – but I wanted to make my own assessment. I also needed to make some initial calculations about how much ketamine I would need for each of the boys, assuming we pressed ahead and got permission to proceed with our plan. I would have to use enough of the drug to ensure each boy stayed unconscious for a good while but not so much that anyone would stop breathing underwater or take too long to recover after the journey out. These were children, after all. I didn't want to drug them any more deeply than I had to. Getting the dosages right would be one of the most difficult judgements I'd have to make: heavier doses for the larger children, smaller doses for the little ones. Size mattered, but there'd still be plenty of guesswork involved.

I also wanted to scope out a precise location for my make-do operating theatre. And I was eager to make friends with the Thai Navy SEALs who had been caring for the boys and the Army medic leading the team, Dr Pak Loharnshoon. Several people had mentioned him, sounding impressed, and I wanted to meet him. We would need the military doctor and his men as allies who could explain to the children in Thai what was about to happen to them, and do it in a way that wouldn't make them freak out or refuse to cooperate.

When Craig and I reached the bottom of the hill, two of the boys had already scampered down to meet us. They must have been the greeting party. The others were still up on the ledge. That slope looked bloody steep to me. It was muddy and slippery and wet. Not that the kids seemed to mind. They were light, and their bare feet were tiny. They dug their toes into the mud and never lost their balance as they trotted down that hill.

As we scrambled up the slope behind them, slipping and sliding and lurching about, their sure-footedness made us feel even more like the middle-aged men we kept being reminded we were. In our partial defence, we had on wetsuit booties, and the boys did not.

'Take shoes off! Take shoes off!'

Some kind people – the British divers? the Thai SEALs? – had installed a rope to steady the climb, which helped a little, but we were puffing and panting and still made fools of ourselves. The kids found the whole thing hilarious.

Headlights came on as we reached the top. Some of the kids were curled up in space blankets. I felt a little like we had invaded their secret camp site. We might have woken a couple of them. But there was no mistaking the thrill in the air. They were delighted to see us, and we were happy to be there.

After we finally got to the top, the boys came over to greet us, bowing and smiling as they made the traditional gesture known as the *wai* – palms together, chin to thumb, as if praying. A couple of the SEALs came to greet us too. We were all bowing and smiling and shaking hands – firm, solid grips all around – when a voice came out of the darkness, clear and strong.

'Hello there.'

The voice belonged to a fit young Thai man with a close-cropped military haircut and a hundred-watt smile. He was Dr Pak – the Royal Thai Army doctor (and lieutenant colonel) supervising the Navy medical team. Besides the Navy SEAL course, we would discover, Pak had completed just about every other training program the Thai military had to offer and was certified for Airborne, Recon, Special Forces, Rangers, Commandos, Para-jumpers and the Queen's Guard. If the Thai military did it, chances are Pak did it too – and might well be the chief instructor for next year's course. He also commanded the Army's 3rd Medical Battalion in Nakhon Ratchasima province, north-east of Bangkok. Put it like this: if I had to be trapped in a cave with no certain release date, I'd definitely want Dr Pak looking after me. The man oozed calm and confidence. He had a physician's caring demeanour and a military officer's complete-the-mission attitude.

The doctor's English wasn't perfect, but it was good enough to communicate and far superior to our non-existent Thai. We spoke slowly, and so did he. 'I'm Harry,' I said. 'This is Craig.' I explained that I was a doctor from Australia and that we were eager to learn about the health of the boys.

Pak seemed happy to oblige. 'Overall,' he said, 'they are in far better condition than I expected. They are all fully conscious. Some minor concerns, but no serious issues. I would say all of them are healthy.'

Amazing.

It was much the same report we'd got from the British divers. Now a physician was saying it too. Given what these boys had been through, could they really be in such terrific shape?

Before we discussed that further, Pak showed us around the camp site, which was now being shared by all seventeen of them – the twelve boys, Coach Ekk and the four members of the Thai military. Conditions were still rough, but they'd improved, the doctor said, as food and other supplies were brought in. Along with the blankets and the torches, there was now a ready store of fruit drinks, energy bars and US Army MREs. No more drinking the questionable cave water. That had been replaced by plastic bottles of fresh water, and a filtration pump brought in by the Thais.

As we spoke with Pak, several of the boys lingered nearby, listening to our conversation, though I don't believe many of them could understand more than a few words. Then one boy, who seemed particularly friendly, approached and spoke to us in English.

'How are you? My name is Adul. What is your name? Welcome to our home in the cave.'

When I praised his English, Adul said he also knew Thai, Burmese, Mandarin and Wa, a language spoken near the border between Myanmar and China. 'I translate for the others if you like,' he said.

Now, that could come in handy.

I returned my attention to Pak. He became animated talking about Ekk, how the team's young assistant coach had led and calmed the boys. 'He is a strong and soothing influence,' the Thai doctor said.

Ekk had told him that on the first two nights they'd been stuck in the cave, emotions ran dangerously high. The boys were crying. They were visibly upset. Several of them seemed certain they would never see their families or friends again. But the coach had called on his training as a novice monk. He led the boys in group meditation, which they happily participated in, partly because he'd invited them to, and partly to ease the boredom of the cave. That seemed to have calmed the boys, and brought the team together and lowered the tension for everyone, Pak said.

The youngest boy, Titan, was terribly scared of the darkness. Ekk kept a special eye on him each night. Though there was zero natural light in the cave, just the torches and the dim glow of the boys' watches, it seemed that their own diurnal rhythms did still make them feel more sleepy at 'night'.

At Coach Ekk's direction, Pak said, the boys had dug a hole into the wall of the cave. It went a good three or four metres. 'The coach didn't really think they could crawl all the way to safety,' Pak said with a smile. 'But he understood it would give them hope, and something to keep them occupied. They needed both of those.'

From their earliest hours in the cave, Pak told us, the coach had done everything he could think of to find a way out. The attempt he'd made on the first night they were trapped was especially valiant.

Ekk had tied a rope around his waist, handing the other end to three of the older boys – Tee, Adul and Night. The coach then climbed into the water, swimming as far as he could in hope of finding an underwater passage. They had a signal worked out in advance.

'If I run out of breath and I can't go any further, I will pull the rope two times. Two times. Then you must pull me back as quickly as you can.'

Now, *that* was a bold plan. Craig and I were amazed at such ingenuity and bravery. But that was only half the tale.

'If I do not pull on the rope,' the young coach had told the boys, 'you will know that I have passed safely through the opening. If I can make it, everybody can.'

The boys had smiled at that, Pak said. Their coach had a game plan.

Ekk held the rope tightly. He stepped into the murky water and waded into the current, which, he told Pak, had been surprisingly stiff. He took a deep breath, the deepest breath he could, filling his lungs with air. He put his head into the water, then pulled himself into the flooded passages with his hands and his feet. He didn't swim exactly. He pulled himself underwater. He could feel the hard rock above his head and soft sand at his toes. He couldn't see anything. The opening was smaller than he had imagined. But he was skinny, and he thought he could fit through.

Ekk kept moving as fast and far as he was able to, constantly bumping against the rocks. When he could go no further, when he felt almost out of air, Ekk knew he had to turn back.

Craig and I hadn't interrupted Pak at all. The story was truly riveting. Ekk's extraordinary attempt to save the boys was an incredible window into what they'd already gone through. Then came the climax.

Unable to hold his breath underwater any longer, Ekk gave the rope two strong pulls and held on tightly. The boys didn't hesitate. Frantically, they hauled him in. He was back with them in just a few seconds. By then, he was gasping for air.

'That way won't work,' Ekk told the boys reluctantly. 'We will find a new way. That is what we will do.'

Bloody hell! I thought.

'To me,' the doctor added, 'Coach Ekk is almost a martyr.'

The young man hadn't just inspired the boys and kept them focused – he'd been willing to risk his life for them.

I looked around, trying to find him among the boys, but I couldn't. At twenty-five, Coach Ekk was a decade older than some of his players, but good luck picking him out of the group. There wasn't much difference between him and some of the older boys. We'd been warned about this by Rick and John, who said the assistant coach looked so young that he could almost pass for a teenager.

I'm not sure where the *almost* came from.

With the camera mounted on my helmet, I shot some video of the boys, waving, smiling, saying hello to their parents and going about their business in the cave. They were all so cheerful and upbeat, it was easy to forget they were stranded in a situation that could very well have cost them their lives and might still. It was almost like they were sending home greetings from school camp.

I had brought along several messages with me in a waterproof pouch. One was a letter from a high-ranking Navy commander to Dr Pak and the SEAL team. I assumed it was a note of encouragement or appreciation or some specific instructions for them. Since the letter was in Thai, I couldn't have read it if I'd tried to. I handed it to Pak, who read it carefully and then passed it on to the other men.

After they'd finished with that, I gave Pak a stack of letters that the boys' families had sent in with us, which within twenty-four hours would be quoted verbatim in the media all around the world. These were the parents' responses to the notes that the boys had sent out the previous day with Jason and Chris.

The boys began to read.

Dear Mark, know that Mummy is waiting for you in front of the cave. I miss you, and please don't feel bad. Mother Hom loves you a lot, and please take good care of yourself.

Dear Biw, Daddy and Mummy miss you. Love you always.

The messages alternated between optimism and heartbreak. But in the brief back-and-forth, you could clearly hear the boys trying to calm their parents and the parents trying to calm the boys. Without a doubt, these children were loved.

Dear Nick, please take care of yourself. Daddy and Mummy are waiting for you. – Father Be, Mother Nang and Nong Bonus.

I didn't know who these people were, but I'll bet Nick was delighted hearing from them.

On every page were little snatches of these families' lives. In the note from his parents, Night's postponed birthday came up again.

Dad and Mum are waiting to arrange your birthday party. Please get out soon, and stay healthy. Mummy knows that you can do it. And you must not be too worried about it. Daddy and Mummy, as well as Grandfather, Grandmother and all the relatives, are supporting you always. Daddy and Mummy love you so much. – Father Boon, Mother O.

One note explained that Mick's grandfather couldn't write properly, so someone had helped him to draft a few lines.

Dear Nong Mick, Grandfather Lek is waiting at the cave's entrance. Grandfather Lek hopes that Mick gets really healthy, and Mick must not be afraid of anyone's condemning him. Grandfather Lek is never angry at you. Grandfather Lek loves Mick always. – Grandfather Lek.

Since Tee's and Dom's parents both had to leave the cave site temporarily to look after their businesses, they had asked a social worker to write notes for them.

Tee and Dom, dads and mums wish you safety. The mental health team told us that your dads and mums have strong health. We wish you strong spirit and to come out. We are waiting for you at the cave's entrance.

Tern's mother wrote a note to all of the boys:

Dear every children, Now every parent is waiting and supporting you. We are not angry at you. Please, take good care of yourselves and cover up with blankets. It's cold, and I'm worried about you boys. You will be out in a short time. Daddy Sak and Mother Ae are waiting for you. – Patchanee Takhamsong (Mother Ae)

Like their fourteen-year-old son, Adul's parents were not Thai Buddhists but stateless Christians, followers of the Baptist faith, and they told him they missed him and were praying for him:

> Father and Mother want to see your face. Father and Mother pray for you and your friends in order to see you soon. After you leave the cave, we want you to say thank you to every official. We want you to trust in God. No worries, Father and Mother will be waiting until you come out.

Like many others, Adul's parents added an extra note of support for the team's assistant coach:

> Thank you for taking care of the children, and leading the children to safety in the times of staying in the dark. Return to the chest of father and mother in the outside. We are waiting outside with love and care too.

Titan's mum also included a shout-out to the coach in her note to her son:

> Titan, be strong. I love you. I'm caring about you. I'm cheering you up! I'm waiting for you in front of the cave. Bring all the boys, Ekk.

Note's and Pong's parents took a similar approach, sprinkled with parental concern.

> Dear Note, Father and Mother are waiting. Take good care of yourself. Father Neung and Mother Dao miss you a lot.

Please tell Coach Ekk not to be too worried. Mother is not angry at him. – Rattanadao Chantapoon

Dear Pong, please take care of your health and stay strong. Father, Mother and everyone are waiting outside to welcome you back to us safely. I would like to thank you, Coach Ekk, for taking care of our twelve children. Coach, please don't be worried. Every parent thanks you for taking care of our children. Daddy and Mummy are waiting to welcome you. – Father Chai and Mother Orn

Coach Ekk's aunt also wrote. She started out like many of the other relatives, but she also reminded her nephew that the boys and their families all loved him and didn't blame him for the ordeal, and that he should please stay strong:

I'm waiting for you in front of the cave. Don't worry too much. Take care of yourself. No one blames you. I urge you to keep fighting. I'm cheering you up. I miss you. No one blames you. Many people are giving you moral support. Keep fighting. I love you. Bring all the boys out. Keep fighting.

Lest there be any doubt about the parents' feelings towards Coach Ekk, several others wrote to him directly, mixing their concern for their children with encouragement for the young man:

Dear Coach Ekk, the parents of every children have asked you to take care of our children. Please, don't blame yourself for this. We want you to rest assured that every parent is not upset or angry at you, and everybody understands and supports you. Thank you very much for taking care of our children. You went into the cave with our children, and you must get out with them. Take our children (and yourself) out with safety. We are waiting in front of the cave.

When the boys were finished reading, it was obvious what an uplifting experience it had been for them to receive these letters. I knew how relieved the parents had been, receiving the notes that Jason and Chris brought out on Friday. I wanted to keep this correspondence going. I figured we might as well give it another round. If the boys wrote replies, Craig and I could carry the notes back out with us.

I passed around a couple of pads. 'Write something,' I said. 'Write something to your parents.'

With some quick translation from Adul and Pak, the boys began scribbling again.

If anything, our short visit with the boys seemed to have them energised. I was happy that they were happy, but it was still strange. Did they understand what terrible danger they were in? Did they know that even those planning to rescue them lacked confidence in the rescue plan? So much smiling in the face of so much peril.

I ran Pak through a basic health survey. The boys, who'd gone entirely without food for nine days and had been subsisting on brought-in rations ever since, all looked super-thin to me. Maybe not as emaciated as some of the most sensational media coverage had implied, but very thin.

'Do any of them have diarrhoea?'

'Is anyone vomiting?'

'Any of them seem particularly weak?'

'Do any have skin irritations that you're worried about?'

'Coughing? Chest infections?'

'There is some coughing,' Pak said. But with a couple of minor exceptions, he answered every other question with an unequivocal *no*.

'They're all good,' he said. 'Morale is high. Things have improved very much since the boys got food. The food is all from America. Steaks. Pasta. Beans. Crackers. They never ate this kind of food before. They really like it!'

I could hear a couple of coughs in the dim light of the cave. Moist coughs, I noticed. That could mean a minor chest cold, or it could mean full-blown pneumonia. Hard to say. Without a proper examination, I had no way of knowing for sure.

Before we came into the cave, I had asked a Thai doctor to help me write a short summary of the rescue plan, as clear and simple as we could make it. Enough to lay out the basics for the boys but not so much as to alarm anyone.

'I have something I'd like you to read out loud,' I said to Pak. 'It's in Thai. It describes a plan for rescuing the boys. Would you read this to them? I want them all to know what will be happening, how we will try to get them out. I don't want anyone to be surprised. We are hoping to start tomorrow.'

I handed Pak the paper. He summoned all the boys, who gathered around him as he read. The first and only words I recognised were 'Dr Harry' and 'Dr Craig'. But as he read on, a horrible thought occurred to me. *I really hope he doesn't stop halfway through this letter and blurt out to everyone: 'You've got to be kidding! You're going to do what? Sedate them and dive them out underwater? This is madness. You know it'll be a death sentence for every one of them.'*

Fine if the Thai military officials wanted to have that discussion privately with Craig and me. I could deal with that. But I definitely didn't want him making a fuss in front of these children. Goodness knows how badly they might be spooked. It would put them in the worst possible frame of mind, just when we needed their cooperation, as the rescue was set to begin.

But Pak did no such thing. About halfway through, he shot me a glance, perfectly businesslike, and then read on.

I could only imagine what he was thinking. He had every right to. *You guys must be crazy. What medical book did you get this one from? All these experts from around the world! Is this the best that you can do?*

I probably agreed with most of that. We *were* crazy to contemplate such a plan. You wouldn't find anything like it in a medical book – we'd dreamed it up ourselves. But it was the best we could do – it was the only real option.

Pak just kept reading.

Though I couldn't understand what he was saying, that didn't matter at all. I already knew the plan. I was far more interested in the boys' reactions. What did they think?

And as the boys took in Pak's words, what was going through their minds?

He read.

They listened.

I watched.

I looked from boy to boy, from face to face, for some kind of sign.

It was only then that I really started to suspect just how tough and resilient these kids were – or how keen they were to get out of there.

Many of them were nodding.

Several smiled.

A couple of them gave the thumbs-up sign.

Not one of them looked the slightest bit like he was going to whimper or cry or collapse to the ground in hysterics. They all just took it on board with a shrug: *Yep, sounds like an excellent plan.*

None of them looked at all afraid.

These kids were prepared to do anything, whatever it took, to get out of this cave.

'When you wake up, you will be outside the cave.' That's what Pak had told the boys at the end of his presentation, as I'd find out later. The Thai doctor on the outside had written that last line a little differently. 'You will wake up in the hospital,' he wrote. Apparently, Pak had decided that ending that way might be too frightening for the boys. So he did a little editing on the fly.

It amazed me how natural Pak seemed with the boys. Though he was obviously a high-ranking military officer, he didn't come off as the least bit intimidating. Maybe it was the doctor in him – or the dad. Even before he told me, I knew Pak had to be a father.

'You've got a good way with these kids,' I told him.

'Thank you,' he said. 'They are good children. They make my job easier. Do you have children, Dr Harry?'

'My wife and I have three,' I said. 'But they're older than these little blokes.'

'I have one,' he said. 'My little boy. When I look at these boys, the smaller ones especially, I can't help it, I see my son. What if something happened to him?'

'Did he know you were coming here?'

'My wife, she knew,' Pak said. 'I told her I would be home in two or three days.'

'I think you're going to be late for dinner,' I said.

'Very late,' he agreed. 'I hope I have not given her too many reasons to worry.'

Before Craig and I said our goodbyes and headed back out of the cave for the night, we had some practical instructions for Pak to follow. If the plan earned final approval from the Thai authorities, we would need him to help prepare the boys for their sedation and the journey out. Prepare them without frightening them.

'We expect to be back tomorrow at midday,' I told Pak. 'Please fast six children from six a.m.,' I continued. 'No food or drink after six. When I call for the first child, I want you to give him an alprazolam tablet to make him feel a bit sleepy and relaxed before the dive. We'll have some more wetsuits for them – masks, cylinders, everything they'll need for the journey.'

I said that I would wait in the water at the base of the steep slope for each boy to be brought down. After a last-minute medical assessment, I would inject the boy in the thigh with a dose of atropine to decrease saliva production, a standard pre-surgical precaution that would be especially important this time to keep all air passages clear and prevent the boy from drowning in his own saliva. As the atropine took effect, I would inject a dose of ketamine, which would render the boy unconscious within five minutes or so. With the help of one of the British divers, we would strap on the diving mask and attach a scuba tank to the boy's chest with rubber bungee cords. Once sedated, each child would be guided out by one of the world's most renowned cave divers, Rick, John, Jason, Chris or one of their other colleagues. Dived out, swum out or carried through cave passages, however the terrain dictated. Breathing steadily. Unable to panic. Being delivered safely to the field hospital outside. The child's condition would be monitored as closely as the divers could manage along the way, focusing most on the depth of sedation. At the earliest sign of consciousness, the young patient would be given a top-up shot of ketamine as needed.

Pak seemed to have no difficulty grasping any of this. I couldn't tell where he stood at this point: was the plan brilliant or crazy or bold, or, as I saw it, some combination of all three?

Maybe Pak was just happy that some other doctor was making this impossible call. Whatever the reason, he seemed to be on board.

'I will help however I can,' he said.

I told him I was deeply grateful, and we most definitely needed his assistance.

I said we wouldn't be able to get all twelve boys plus Coach Ekk out in a single day. We figured each trip would take three or four hours, and we needed generous spacing between them. We would try for six boys the first day, but getting everyone out could take two or three days.

'Come up with an order,' I told Pak. 'Let us know which of the boys you'd like us to send out first. Discuss it with the coach. Discuss it with the boys. You decide.'

My preference, though I didn't push it, was to send a couple of the strongest ones out first, giving ourselves the greatest chance of early success. That way, maybe we could build some confidence while we honed our medical and diving moves.

'We will make an order,' Pak promised.

I really felt like I had found an important partner, when and where I needed one most, in this young Thai military doctor. I told Pak that I knew the boys had been in good hands, and that together we would work to get everyone out.

He smiled at that. 'Harry,' he asked, 'what do you enjoy doing when you are not here?'

As I often do, I blurted out the first thing that popped into my mind. 'I like drinking beer.'

'That's good,' Pak answered without missing a beat. 'When we are all out, we will go drink a Thai beer.'

We spoke different languages. We lived in very different lands. But there was something deeply comforting in knowing that Pak and I could both enjoy a beer.

As Craig and I said our goodbyes for the evening, all the boys were smiling and waving at us.

None of them knew what we knew: that despite our seeming confidence and our studied nonchalance, the mission that we'd soon be launching was anything but foolproof. Those of us who had devised it knew that better than anyone.

As we strapped on our masks and our tanks and climbed back into the water for the long dive out, Rick's words echoed inside my head.

'You're going to dive to the end of the cave,' he'd said the day he'd called me at the hospital. 'You're going to see these kids. They're all looking healthy and happy and smiley. Then you're going to swim away and probably leave them all to die. Be mindful of that before you say yes with too much enthusiasm.'

I had tried to, but here we were.

The boys looked healthy and happy and smiley, and I couldn't say with any confidence what was next for them.

'See you tomorrow,' I said, with my own studied cheerfulness. 'Big day ahead.'

I could only hope that would turn out to be true.

13

General Assembly

Harry

It was half past seven when we climbed out of the water and half past eight when we stepped out of the cave. It was after nine by the time we returned to the British camp headquarters and got to speak with the Brits and the Americans. I was eager to hear how their swimming-pool run-through had gone.

'Brilliantly,' Rick beamed.

They'd tested the bungee cords and the cylinder placement. They made adjustments to the face masks and the buoyancy weights. They got all the gear right where they wanted it, performing flawlessly in the pool. And nothing bad had happened to any of the teenage volunteers, even when the Brits passed them from diver to diver without ever coming up for air. Everyone got safely out of the pool.

Jamie Brisbin had been key here. One of the pararescue guys with the 31st Rescue Squadron of the US Air Force, he was also an equipment whiz. He'd stripped all the face masks, tweaked and reassembled them, securing the seals and adjusting the airflow to perfectly accommodate the special challenges of the cave environment. This came as no surprise to Craig and me. We'd got to know Jamie way back in 2009, when he travelled to Australia as a Rolex Scholar with the Our World-Underwater Scholarship Society. His adventures that year included joining us on an exploration of Cocklebiddy Cave. We were surprised when he showed up at the cave in Thailand – he'd interrupted his family holiday in Kyoto, Japan, to be here.

'You thought I would miss this?' he asked.

Based on the pool experiment, Rick did say he wanted to make one last adjustment: binding the kids' wrists behind their backs, perhaps with cable ties and spring-loaded carabiners, and tying their ankles together with bungees. It was important for the boys to be as streamlined as possible while the divers ferried them through the cave's restricted passages and narrow openings. 'We don't want to bang anybody around unnecessarily,' Rick said.

The way he described it, we'd be wrapping the anaesthetised children into tight little packages before shipping them out of the cave – our own underwater FedEx, more or less. We wouldn't be asking much from the unconscious boys but to keep breathing and not to cause any trouble along the way. These precautions, Rick said, would reduce the chance of a stray arm or leg or other body part getting caught on an obstruction in the water, or injured in some other way. And if one of the boys woke up from the anaesthesia, he'd still be safely constrained.

Since the British divers had made the trip into the cave several times already, they didn't have too much to learn from us about the inside of the cave. They did want to hear our impressions of Dr Pak and the boys, though. I told Rick I could now understand what he meant about meeting all those smiling children and then saying goodbye, not knowing what the future had in store for them.

'Sobering,' I allowed.

We were still waiting for the green light from the Thais, but in the meantime Rick wrote up a tentative line-up of divers for the next day, including what roles everyone would play. The first change was that we were no longer going to attempt six rescues on day one. That seemed like too many. In addition, only four really suitable full face masks had been identified that day in the pool. Instead, Rick and the other three most experienced British divers – John, Chris and Jason – would be the ones ferrying the first four boys out of the cave, each diver responsible for one boy. Other divers, including Craig, would be stationed at strategic locations inside the cave, assessing the boys' condition, keeping things moving and, when needed, giving top-ups of ketamine to any boy who seemed to be waking from his drug-induced slumber.

Two European divers, Claus Rasmussen of Denmark and Mikko Paasi of Finland, would join Craig in chamber 8. Ivan Karadzic, also from Denmark, and Canadian Erik Brown would be meeting the boys in chamber 6. They would help and support the mission in any way needed.

Craig and Rick would have special duties, a bit different from the other divers. Craig would give each boy a thorough check-up after the initial leg of the perilous underwater dive. That would be our very first chance to see if the plan could possibly work or not. Could we really dive a sedated child through a flooded cave and not kill him on the way? Craig would be the first one to know. With his years as a veterinary surgeon, he had the skill and experience to make this crucial judgement. He knew ketamine. He knew respiration. He knew vital signs and what they might mean. Though his practice focused on animals, almost all of that knowledge applies just as well to humans. Craig was perfectly suited to the role. It would also allow him to demonstrate directly to all the other divers how to assess the health of the boys along the way and decide whether to give them a further dose.

Rick would have double-duty when the rescue finally began. He would begin the day with Craig, Claus and Mikko in chamber 8. As soon as the first boy came through and Craig completed his field assessment, Rick would swim back to me in chamber 9 and deliver an early progress report. *How did the first leg of the dive go? How does the boy look? What is Craig saying? Did the ketamine dose seem about right? What mistakes could we correct when carrying out extractions 2 to 13?* That way, Craig's assessment wouldn't just help the first boy. It would be a learning tool for all of us. I would wait to hear back from Rick before sedating and sending out the second boy.

So what were we forgetting? Would we have enough divers in the cave? There were a lot of moving parts here, and they would call for the help of many hands. Rick asked who else I knew.

'There's a couple of divers from Australia we could get, and it would be quicker to get them up here, obviously, in terms of travel time,' I said. But given the bureaucratic obstacles we faced in getting Craig here, I couldn't promise anything. 'I can see the DFAT guys having kittens at the very idea of asking for two more,' I said.

'Don't worry,' Rick said. 'We'll get a few more of our guys.' He mentioned Jim Warny, Connor Roe and Josh Bratchley, rising stars a decade or two younger than we were. 'They'll be fine, and they'll be here,' Rick said to John. 'They'll be up for the adventure. Just get them.'

*

While we'd been honing our rescue plan, Elon Musk had been busy too. The billionaire tech entrepreneur was back home in Bel Air, California, posting updates on Twitter.

'Some good feedback from cave experts in Thailand,' he tweeted on Saturday night, 7 July, Thai time, to his 26 million followers. 'Iterating with them on an escape pod design that might be safe enough to try. Also building an inflatable tube with airlocks. Less likely to work, given tricky contours, but great if it does.'

It was hard to know exactly who the Tesla founder was 'iterating with' and who was giving him all this 'good feedback'. Anyone we knew with cave experience seemed to be greeting Musk's escape pod and inflatable tube with raised eyebrows, often followed by a curt: 'That'll never work.' But high-profile creative geniuses aren't easily discouraged, especially those sitting high on the *Forbes* rich list with a net worth hovering around US$20 billion. Musk was not deterred.

A bit later on Saturday, he tweeted again. 'Got more great feedback from Thailand. Primary path is basically a tiny, kid-size submarine using the liquid oxygen transfer tube of Falcon rocket as hull. Light enough to be carried by 2 divers, small enough to get through narrow gaps. Extremely robust.' And then: 'Continue to be amazed by the bravery, resilience & tenacity of kids & diving team in Thailand. Human character at its best.'

In the days and weeks to come, Musk's attempts to insert himself into the drama at the cave would become a source of debate, controversy and ridicule, resulting in plenty of media coverage, not to mention a bitter lawsuit. But for now, the actual rescue preparations were proceeding entirely without him.

*

Back to reality.

Nothing could happen without the approval of the Thai government. Everyone understood that. As the plan slowly came together, it was Rick and John and the Americans who had been taking primary responsibility for meeting with the Thais. And meeting with them. And meeting with them. Mostly, Craig and I were able to sidestep it all. But after our divers' briefing late on Saturday, I got called in for a thorough grilling by the full Thai hierarchy – political, medical and military. They seemed to have a lot of questions. The medical people spoke first.

'How did you choose the drugs?'

'Why these dosages?'

'Why alprazolam? Why not something longer acting?'

I calmly explained my thinking. I said I thought these were the best choices, but I was happy for other options to be proposed and considered. I didn't want to argue with anyone. I wanted consensus.

It was a crowded room. Besides the Thai government people and the British divers and Craig and me, we had the American military, some Chinese military, a couple of people from the AFP and some others who came from I-wasn't-sure-where. The language barrier made all this cumbersome. I spoke in English. The Thais spoke in Thai and English. Other people interpreted.

The Thai officials had a right to be sceptical. They didn't know us. Why should they trust us to handle this job?

Think about it. We're a mob of uninspiring-looking middle-aged men. We've jetted into your country from around the world. We have all this dodgy looking, partially homemade dive equipment, and we're covered in mud. And we're telling you, 'Don't use your own military. We can handle this.'

If you're a Thai general, what do you do?

It may be that the Thai Navy SEALs, who'd had virtually no cave-diving experience, weren't fighting any of this. After the death of Saman Gunan, they may well have decided, *Let the foreigners handle it*. But the decision was clearly in the hands of the generals. After a while, one of them sat up straight in his chair – even straighter than he had been sitting – and looked directly at me.

'With this rescue,' he asked in a low, gravelly voice, 'can you guarantee success?'

'Absolutely not,' I answered. 'We can pretty much guarantee that it *won't* be a total success. But there's no alternative.'

He didn't ask anything else after that.

It didn't seem like we were going to get an answer immediately. But I was heartened by the fact that no one seemed to be pushing any alternative schemes. 'Assuming we are going in the morning,' I said finally, 'we do need the ketamine prepared.'

I knew we had enough alprazolam and atropine to ease the boys' anxiety and dry their mouths. But I told the Thai medical people exactly what ketamine doses I wanted and what size syringes. In my mind, I had divided the boys into two groups: the forty-kilo kids and the fifty-kilo kids. I was basing the dosages around that. The fifty-kilo group would get 250 milligrams of ketamine to start with. The forty-kilo kids would get 200 milligrams. I knew I could vary the doses to suit the kids' more precise weights, but that would make things a whole lot more complicated for the divers. I needed to keep the process as simple as possible for them.

Picking the right top-up for intramuscular ketamine was anybody's guess. Nobody usually does intramuscular ketamine top-ups. If a patient started rousing in the operating theatre, you'd already have inserted an IV, and tiny doses would be slowly titrated in. But I needed an answer. 'Let's say a half-dose,' I declared.

'That'll be about right.' None of this is standard medical practice, because there was nothing standard about this situation.

In my entire career, I think I had given one person a dose of intramuscular ketamine, a massive psychiatric patient in an emergency department. I'd jabbed him in the leg like I was darting a dangerous animal and run away as quickly as I could, waiting for him to drop. And I'd never done an intramuscular top-up. We were making it up as we went along.

Even without formal approval, the Thai medical people got to work – just in case, I guess. All of this, from the initial dose to the top-ups, involved a little bit of science. I tried not to let on just how much guesswork was also involved.

14

Hard Choices

Craig

As well as we were able to, we had prepared ourselves for success.

Our rescue plan was as solid as we could make it, whatever limitations it might still have. Harry seemed comfortable with his makeshift operating theatre – not perfect, but good enough. I felt confident about the medical assessment I'd give each boy in chamber 8, and about the pass-off strategy we'd settled on too. Harry had promised to give the other divers a lesson in the morning to teach them how to inject ketamine, and I figured they'd be okay. I wouldn't want them performing complex surgery, but giving injections isn't too hard. Even the sceptical Thai authorities appeared to be leaning in our direction. If they really hated the idea, they wouldn't have let the medical staff count out the pills and load the syringes with ketamine. But there was one remaining question, and you couldn't call it trivial. It was truly a matter of life and death.

What would we do if the kids began to die?

It was a brutal question, but also unavoidable. It was the question that Heather and Fiona had asked before we'd even left Australia.

It had been haunting Harry and me from the moment we began to accept that anaesthesia was really the only practical option. If kids started dying, would we keep pressing forwards? Or would we stop and reconsider, knowing that we'd already considered every option we could think of? How many dead boys would it take until we said *no more*? One? Two? Five? How many? And if we abandoned the plan we had settled on, what alternatives did we have?

If you think these are easy questions, you haven't given them enough thought.

There was, after all, a limited range of outcomes here. It was possible – unlikely but *possible* – that the plan would work perfectly and everyone would survive. Children and divers both. If that happened, the only question would be . . . beer, wine or hard liquor – what would we toast ourselves with at the celebratory bash? But on the other hand, what if it didn't go so well, as we feared it might? What if the first boy died on the way out of the cave? Would we send another boy after him? What if we did, and he died too? Could we bring ourselves to keep sending more boys on the perilous underwater journey?

It was tempting to avoid thinking about this, because the prospect was so disturbing. But Harry and I needed to prepare ourselves for this very real possibility.

I knew that Harry and Fiona had wrestled with the prospect of failure before he and I met up in Thailand. He'd told me that she had raised the thorny question of what it might mean for him to be known as the doctor who killed the Thai soccer kids. That would be a heavy burden to carry through life. Heather had raised her own dark fears about the potential for disaster. But if kids started dying while the operation was still under way, what would we actually *do*? Pack up and go home?

This was anything but hypothetical. It was as real as real could be. Both Harry and I and everyone else involved in this plan fully expected that at least some of these children would die. We all had the same scenarios looping through our heads: we would start on the first day with live children inside the cave. By the time the day was over, we would most likely be swimming dead children through the cave. This was never far from our minds, even as we pressed the Thais and others to give us the go-ahead.

'I have to tell you,' Harry said to me in the DFAT van as we headed for the hotel that night, 'if the first couple die, I might have to stop. I'm not sure I'll be able to keep sending children to their deaths, even if we're still convinced.'

This was a difficult thing for Harry to say. He's a very practical and realistic person, and as a doctor he gets a special kick out of working in the most life-threatening crises imaginable, ready to do his best no matter how dreadful the circumstances or how daunting the odds. But doctors are supposed to save people, not kill them.

'I want you to know there's a limit to how far I can go,' he said.

'I get that,' I told him.

In a very real sense, Harry and I would be the ones making the call, Harry especially. Depending on what happened with the first few children, he would have to decide whether or not to anaesthetise the boys who were waiting to go next. Without Harry, nothing else could go forward.

'You know, I'm still not convinced any of this is going to work,' he reminded me, not that I needed reminding.

He paused, struggling to articulate the fear he hadn't been able to shake. 'It could be like I'm euthanising these boys.'

As we talked this through, I realised that we felt a bit differently about the fundamental choice we faced. Harry was grappling with the idea that he might be setting out to kill his patients, while I was focused on our lack of alternatives. Even though we agreed that the approach we'd be taking put the boys in mortal danger, could we really abandon it if it was still the best option we had?

'Harry,' I said, when I saw the pained look wasn't leaving his face, 'we've gone round and round, and this is the best of all the possible options. We can't leave them in there for months until the monsoon season is over. If we do that, they'll surely die. 'If we bring them out now, there's a chance some will survive. That might give some of them a way out.'

Harry didn't seem convinced.

'So if I accept it's horribly dangerous, then what?' he asked. 'At least if they die this way, they'll die asleep under the water rather than have a painful, lingering death in the cave that might take months? Is that it?'

'It's an impossible choice,' I conceded. 'But this part is up to you. You have to be all right with it, whatever you decide.'

We sat in silence then as the van bounced along the bumpy streets of Mae Sai, each of us lost in thought. Finally, Harry broke the quiet. 'I think I have to go ahead with it,' he said, almost in a whisper, as if he were really talking to himself. 'At least if they drown, they'll be anesthetised. When it happens, they'll be asleep. They won't know anything about it at all.'

I waited a moment, not sure how to answer. 'Look,' I said, 'we reckon we've already thought of every possible plan. If the first one or two kids die, I think we'll still have to push forwards. If there's something obvious going wrong that we can address, we will, but the equation won't have changed. The first one might die and then the next twelve might be successful. The first two might die and the next eleven might be successful. Unless we've got new information, there won't be any reason to change what we're doing. The kids will still be trapped there. We can't just leave them to what we agree is certain death if they stay in the cave. They still deserve the best shot at survival, whatever that is.'

I can't say Harry and I really found an answer to this question. It was probably unresolvable. We ended at what you might call a respectful impasse with reality. We'd been as plain as could be with each other. We had recognised and acknowledged the arguments on both sides. We would face the issue if and when we had to – but we desperately hoped we never would. Until then, it was just a horrible question hanging in the air.

It wasn't the only one, of course. There was also the question of who should be told if the children started to die during the extraction.

Outside the cave, Thai government officials would announce whatever they chose to announce and at whatever speed. That was up to them, and we couldn't control it. But given the constant swarm of foreign media, it was hard to imagine how the news could be kept secret for long. If kids lived or kids died, that would leak out in a hurry. I had no doubt about that. But for me, the more difficult question was this: if children started dying, what should we say, if anything, to the other boys, to the coach and to the Thai Navy SEALs looking after them?

'Your friends Mark and Pong just drowned on their way out of the cave – are you ready to go now?'

Harry would receive a report from me after the first boy had arrived in chamber 8, letting him know when it was safe to send the next one, but we would have no idea of the outcome of the first rescue attempts until the end of the day. There was no real communication from outside the cave. The only way to get a message through was to send it with a cave diver – and all of them would be in the cave already, participating in the rescue. If a boy died after leaving chamber 8, we wouldn't know it until that evening. If our estimates were right, and each dive took three or four hours, we'd already have sent the next unconscious boys on their way, possibly to their deaths. That was chilling to me.

But eventually, we would know. We would know before the second day of the rescue – assuming we were going to proceed.

What then?

Should we tell the other children? Should we tell the SEALs? Should we duck the issue? Should we lie?

I came to a tentative conclusion that surprised me.

Against my better judgement, and despite the high value I have always placed on openness and honesty – I was inclined to lie. I would say to the remaining children, 'Everyone's okay,' even if they weren't.

I couldn't believe I was thinking like this, but I was.

If I had to do that, I knew it would trouble me deeply. But what else could we do? If any of their friends had perished and we had decided to press on, telling the full truth would make things drastically worse for all the remaining boys. And besides, even armed with the truth, what position were they in to judge the best available course? They were children in a vulnerable situation that they had no control over. They lacked experience and full knowledge of the facts. We had both, and it was up to us to make that decision for them.

Harry and I kicked this question back and forth between us. We tried to look at it from all directions, but he ended up in much the same place I did. Reluctantly, he said he might have no real option but to lie. 'I'm not sure I'm actually capable of telling a lie like that,' he said. 'It obviously doesn't feel right. But saying "your friends have died" seems even worse. I just hope we never have to decide. I'd hate to be tested on this.'

Harry and I didn't talk about this with anyone else at the cave, including the British divers. Other people might have been having the same conversation – I don't know. I assume they were. But that's about where we ended up, reluctant but resigned.

There's so much emphasis today on people making informed choices about their own destinies. I believe in that wholeheartedly. I know Harry does too. Where there's uncertainty, people should be given all the information so they can make their own well-informed choices. That concept is at the core of living in a free world. Generally speaking, it's hard to argue against.

Then real life intervenes. A group of children are stranded in a flooded cave. Everyone wants to help them, and everyone has a plan to save them. They can't possibly know which plan is best. All they know is that they want to get out alive.

We forget that sometimes that whole beautiful concept – full disclosure, risk assessment, informed consent – it's not really applicable or desirable for the people who are the victims. Sometimes, somebody just needs to take charge. This time, we would be the ones to assume responsibility – to decide, uncomfortably, on their behalf.

15

Med School

Harry

We heard nothing more from the Thai authorities on Saturday night. They were still weighing their options, it seemed, deciding whether to trust the lives of thirteen young people to a scruffy band of middle-aged foreigners who claimed to have special expertise in diving in and out of water-filled caves.

This would be a big leap for the Thais. They were immensely proud of their armed forces, especially the elite Royal Thai Navy SEALs. Ideally, the SEALs would be handling everything, not just babysitting the children while foreign civilians swooped in to run the rescue. Thailand was getting worldwide media attention it hadn't received in decades. The ruling military junta, a subject of endless controversy since the 2014 coup, would be judged on all of this. Whatever their hesitation, deliberations went on long into the night.

By the time Craig and I headed back to our rooms, we'd still heard nothing more about the Bangkok Hilton and our up-in-the-air diplomatic immunity. If something went wrong in the cave, if one of us screwed up somehow, even if one of the kids died through no fault of our own, would I be held legally responsible? Would I, to use Michael Costa's ominous phrase, 'end up in the Thai judicial system'? Would I be joining Nicole Kidman's tragic character as the Bangkok Hilton's next Aussie inmate?

As I'd requested, Michael hadn't mentioned this possibility since he'd first brought it up on Friday. I'd just assumed we would know something as soon as he did. Whatever conversations were occurring between the Thais and the Australians – or more likely within the Thai regime – we had so many other things to worry about that I hadn't stressed much over this. But there was no telling when an answer might come or whether it would even come at all. Maybe we'd all be taking our chances inside the cave. Craig and I both went to bed late on Saturday with a whole lot unresolved.

It turned out that the question of diplomatic immunity had gone all the way to the top of the Thai government. No obscure Thai bureaucrat was going to decide our fate! When the decision finally came, at 11.53 p.m. that night, it was made by Don Pramudwinai, the nation's minister of foreign affairs. Even then, the news had to tumble through the Thai bureaucracy and down through the Australian diplomatic corps before it got to us: the foreign-affairs minister alerted Sarun Charoensuwan, director general of Thailand's Department of American and South Pacific Affairs, who sent an email to Paul Robilliard, Australia's ambassador to Thailand.

Pursuant to the Australian Embassy's Note No. Pol 47/18 dated 6 July 2018, I wish to inform you that, after consultation among concerned Thai agencies, Foreign Minister Don Pramudwinai has given his approval to grant diplomatic privileges and immunities to Mr Richard James Dunbar HARRIS and Mr Craig Jonathan CHALLEN, who are working with the Thai authorities on the rescue mission at Tham Luang cave in Chiang Rai Province.

Please be informed that the diplomatic privileges and immunities will be granted to the aforementioned Australian nationals on condition that the Thai authorities have chosen the sedation method in support of the said rescue mission.

Michael Costa forwarded the verdict to us at 3.18 a.m., though Craig and I didn't see the overnight email traffic until we woke up on Sunday morning, eager to hear what, if anything, was coming next. 'I will also get in writing that the Thais approved your sedation method,' Michael added in his forwarding note.

Since we hadn't been told yet that the Thais actually *did* approve of our sedation method, I wasn't sure how Michael was going to do that. But given the time stamps on all these emails, the man certainly didn't waste much time sleeping. Maybe he had a way.

When Craig and I got to the Thai medical tent around 8 a.m., we still hadn't received the final word. Was the rescue a goer? Despite no clear answers, all the signs were pointing to yes. Thai nurses and medics had spent the night preparing and labelling syringes – *full dose, half-dose, large boy, small boy* – just as I had asked them to, simple and clear as could be. One of the nurses opened the lids on a pair of large styrofoam eskies. 'All the drugs are in here,' she said. I transferred the loaded syringes into four ziploc bags and then labelled each bag. Then Craig and I headed over to the Brits' head-quarters to meet with all the divers who'd be going into the cave with us, if and when formal permission was received. I had a first-year medical school class to teach.

Anaesthesia 101.

There was no way an initial injection of ketamine was going to last for three or four hours, our best guess at how long it would take a diver to ferry one of the boys out of the cave. Each diver would need to give a top-up dose the moment his boy seemed to be stirring awake. I didn't want one of the kids coming to, thrashing around and drowning himself and the diver who was trying to get him out.

The unscheduled wake-up might happen at one of the designated chamber stops. That would be preferable. But it could just as easily happen underwater in one of the sumps. I needed to get all the divers comfortable enough to give these top-up shots. I knew this would be a stretch for some of them.

These were divers, not doctors. Most of them had never handled a syringe before. Giving a jab is completely routine for a doctor or, especially, a nurse. But for someone without medical training, it can be extremely intimidating. Believe me, I know.

I will never forget the first time I put a needle into someone's arm. I was drunk. As first-year medical students, my classmates and I were asked to perform a little experiment testing blood-alcohol levels. First, each of us downed a couple of beers. In fact, to guarantee a strong positive result, a few of us had snuck off to the university tavern before the session. Then we were told to take a blood sample from our lab partner and test the blood-alcohol level. I was paired with a student who went on to become a highly respected colorectal surgeon. He came from the country and had grown up working on farms, but he absolutely couldn't stand the sight of blood.

He whispered to me, 'I'll faint if I do this.'

'You'll be doing it to *me*,' I reminded him. 'Please don't faint.'

I went first. I focused, steadying my hand and steeling my mind against the alcohol. Then I gulped and slid the needle into my partner's arm. I was terrified. No matter who you are, jabbing a needle into someone's arm for the first time and sucking the blood out is challenging.

Then it was his turn to jab me. He poked the needle into my arm – so far, so good. I think he even hit the vein. But then, *whoa*! He keeled right over and slumped to the floor. I had to reach down and yank the needle out.

I have no idea how he made it through his first surgery rotation, but somehow he did.

I had worked on farms as a teenager, too, and killed sheep by cutting their throats with a knife. I gutted and cleaned them. I'd done the same with kangaroos. By the time I was a med student, I thought I was fairly robust when it came to blood and gore. But I'd still had trouble the first time I had to poke a needle into someone else.

So how would the other divers do? Could we count on them to give the top-up shots when needed? We were all about to learn. I had no idea what to expect from these cave-diving blokes.

I showed them how the syringes were packaged, the different doses for different-sized kids. 'It's the half-doses you'll be working with,' I explained. 'By the time the boys get to you, I'll already have given them the full doses to make them go to sleep.'

I held up one of the syringes and pointed out the little cap on the end. 'That's so it won't leak or get contaminated,' I said. 'What you need to do is remove the cap and put the needle on the end of the syringe. Then, you take the cover off the needle and —' I tried to sound equal parts nonchalant and professorial — 'inject it.'

I could see faces flinching around me, heard them draw in breath, as if a needle had just gone into every diver's arm.

I'd better take this a little more slowly, I thought.

'It all starts with you looking at the kid,' I said. 'If you think he looks like one of the smaller ones, use *this* syringe.' I held up one of the clearly labelled 100s. 'If you think he looks like one of the bigger kids, use *this* syringe.' I waved a 125.

'How many of you have given injections before?' I asked the divers.

Only Claus raised his hand.

He had trained as a remote emergency medical technician and had been with the Red Cross in his native Denmark. 'I've played with needles before,' he said. 'I've done enough first aid to feel like I can do it.'

To one degree or another, the others all expressed concern.

It was time to demonstrate.

I had an empty plastic water bottle, the single-serving kind, and a couple of empty syringes, which I passed out to the guys. 'Okay, everyone,' I said. 'Here are some empty syringes and bungs and caps and needles. Now that you know what all the different pieces are for, I want you to assemble one of these, pretend it's got liquid in it and inject it into this water bottle.'

Really? they seemed to ask without saying a word.

I pressed on.

'I want it to go in at least three-quarters of the length of the needle, then you're going to squeeze the imaginary liquid slowly into the flesh.'

I passed the bottle to the first diver, who slid the needle through the plastic and depressed the plunger at the butt end of the syringe. The injection looked fairly smooth.

'Easy, eh?' I said encouragingly.

He didn't answer. But he did pass the bottle to the next diver, who performed his own injection and passed the bottle on. If there had been water inside that bottle, by now it would have been leaking all over the floor. Everyone had a practice. They seemed to be getting the hang of it fairly quickly. They were sliding through plastic, of course, not human tissue. Mentally, it's a different thing. But these were can-do cave divers, and they all performed better than I expected them to.

The comments trickled in.

'Oh, yeah.'

'That's not so bad.'

'I think I have the feel of it. I can do that.'

We still had to make the leap from water bottle to sedated boy, and that required further explanation.

'The best thing to do,' I said, 'is to inject the outside front quarter of the upper leg, anywhere on the outside thigh between the knee and the hip. Make sure you push the needle in far enough so that you get through the wetsuit. If you inject the drug into the wetsuit, it's not going to work. Don't worry if you go too far and you hit the bone.'

I was rewarded with several noticeable winces.

'Just come back a little and then inject it,' I continued. 'You won't hurt the kid. You won't do any harm. There are no nerves or blood vessels there. Just bung it in and inject it. It will work. This stuff works anywhere you stick it. If you get it in their body, it will work – every time.'

Ketamine, I explained, is an extremely safe drug. 'Don't worry about overdosing the kid,' I said. 'Just make sure you're safe by having the kid quiet at all times. If he looks like he's rousing, give him some more. But don't give them two doses in less than about ten minutes. It takes a few minutes to work. You've got to let the first dose take effect. Apart from that, just go for it.' I looked around to see if everyone seemed comfortable. 'Nothing can possibly go wrong,' I added earnestly.

These divers were practical, tough, pragmatic people. I'm sure they saw right through my exaggerated confidence. But they also seemed happy to be reassured.

The drug, I said, does have its own unique effects. Patients can appear slightly strange while they are sleeping. 'Sometimes,' I said, 'they might be moaning or moving around a little. Sometimes, their eyes are open, even though they're asleep. The brain is still in a sleep mode. On ketamine, the dividing line between asleep and awake can be a little blurry.'

Simple rule of thumb, I told the divers: 'If you're in doubt, if the child is rousing or physically moving to the point of it being a problem, give him more.'

Each child, I predicted, would need two or three doses on the way out.

With that, the lecture was over. That was the extent of Anaesthesia 101.

After my little class, a couple of the divers came up to me with a few last questions about the practicalities of it all. But everyone seemed satisfied. And just in case we got the thumbs-up to rescue anyone, I passed out the first-day batches of ketamine, two or three doses for each diver. Most of the divers seemed comfortable enough.

I had the impression that Claus was deeply affected by the assignment we could soon be taking on, but he didn't seem to want to discuss it. His way of dealing with it was to tell himself: *We have a job to do. Let's get on with it.*

Jason seemed fine to me – he was a bit like Craig: focused and driven. I'm not sure he spent much time weighing his feelings.

I did get a quiet moment alone with John. Of all the divers, he was the only one who expressed genuine disquiet to me about what lay ahead. The prospect of bringing dead children out of the cave was clearly preying on his mind.

'I hope we won't regret this,' he said, as if saying so might help to ward it off.

I'm not saying John was the only one who felt that way. I don't believe he was. But he was the only one willing to own the feeling out loud.

It was just then that we got the final word.

The plan had been approved by the Thai authorities.

The news came with little drama. It was almost anticlimactic. One of the Thai officials told Rick, who told us. No fanfare. No press releases. No uniformed generals talking on TV. Just a message passed along.

It's a go.

We had official permission to enter the cave, sedate the children and dive them out.

It was up to us now.

It was near 10 a.m. We started suiting up and assembling our gear. And off we went to the cave.

IV

Saving

16

Final Prep

Harry

I dived with Jason.

Focused, driven, unstoppable Jason.

He and I went in first, to be followed by Craig and Rick and then the others.

There were too many of us to dive into the cave all together. So we split into pairs. Since I would be anaesthetising the boys and Jason would be diving the first one out, it made sense for the two of us to go in together and first. We had to travel further than any of the other divers would initially, all the way to chamber 9. We needed to be sure that Pak and the SEALs had followed all our instructions and readied the first wave of boys for their long, gruelling, sedated trips out. Fasted them. Dressed them. Prepared them mentally. Confirmed which ones would be up first. And had boy number one shipshape and ready to go.

'I don't know what you were so concerned about,' Jason said to me as we made our way from chamber to chamber, sump to sump, and through a couple of the cave's tighter constrictions. 'You're racing along.'

Jason is such a machine in the water, I was happy I could keep up with him. He seemed to have no anxiety about going first. If anyone could do it, this tough bugger could.

But why did I feel so spent? Had Saturday's dive knocked me around more than I realised? The main event was upon us. Twelve Thai children and their young soccer coach were waiting expect-antly, desperately hoping we could save their lives. The whole world was tuned in. I needed to be at my absolute best. But by the time Jason and I were halfway to chamber 9, I felt cold and shivery – weak as a kitten – pulling myself hand over hand along the rope, trying to get into some sort of rhythm. It was like I was getting the flu.

I really can't afford to blow this, I said to myself.

I had a diving pouch clipped off behind me like a little purse. That's where I had the drugs: the alprazolam for easing the boys' anxiety, the atropine for drying up their saliva and the ketamine to knock them out, plus the syringes and needles I would need to deliver those drugs. Craig, Rick and the others, diving in behind us, would have their own carrying techniques. Some would stash their ketamine top-ups in a wetsuit pocket. Others would use waterproof bags. Along with their own drugs, Rick, Jason, John and Chris would each swim into the cave with an extra cylinder and a full face mask for the boys to use. Those cylinders contained 80 per cent oxygen, a higher percentage than usual, though not the pure oxygen we had originally hoped to use.

Some patients breathe inadequately under anaesthesia. In a normal operating theatre, increased inspired levels of oxygen help keep patients nice and pink. But there was a more urgent reason this time: if a kid began to drown inside the cave, there'd be a much better chance of resuscitating him if he had a high level of oxygen on board. If your body is primed with oxygen, the brain will live longer after your breathing stops. On a high-risk dive like this one, that could mean the difference between brain damage, life and death. Please, no backyard experiments! But with sufficient oxygen and in a slightly cooled, anaesthetised patient, the brain might survive as long as ten minutes, twice the normal time.

I hoped we'd never need that extra margin of safety, but we'd sure be grateful to have it if we did. Unfortunately, the Thai Navy personnel who were filling the oxygen cylinders had somehow managed to destroy all the booster pumps that would send gas from a large low-pressure oxygen cylinder into the smaller high-pressure ones. In other words, we couldn't fill the tanks to sufficient pressure with pure oxygen. A bit more than three-quarters full was as high as we could go. So we topped off the boys' cylinders with regular air to create sufficient pressure, about 200 bar, and told ourselves that would have to do. It meant that the cylinders had 80 per cent oxygen in them rather than 100 per cent, but that was close enough.

Anyway, I wasn't feeling any better as Jason and I swam into chamber 8. I was lightheaded and a little nauseated. We lingered there as Craig and Rick arrived. 'It's almost like the gas I've been breathing isn't clean,' I said to the others. But Jason looked okay. So did Craig and Rick. At least so far. And I had no time to fret about it. We had work to do. All we could do was swim on.

The boys noticed us before we noticed them. They had an excellent view from atop their ledge. When they caught sight of Jason and me, they seemed just as hyped as they had the day before. More so, actually. As we approached, I could hear their chattering voices. This was a big day for us. It was so much bigger for them. If any of the boys felt nervous about the death-defying journey ahead, I didn't sense it in the chamber's dank air. I'll tell you what I was feeling: like we'd just swum into Christmas morning, and I was Santa Claus.

Jason and I took our gear off and laid it on the small beach across the water from the hill where the boys were. Then we swam over to the base of the slope with the cylinder, the full face mask and the pouch filled with pills, needles and syringes. I found a rope over to the right, where I clipped my little goodie bag so it would stay out of the unsanitary water. It was then that I looked up to see Dr Pak coming down the mud slide from above.

'G'day,' I called out to him. He was not as sure on his feet as the boys were – who was? – but definitely steadier than Craig or I had been the day before. Dr Pak, I was beginning to realise, always looked in command whatever he was doing, wherever he was. The thought did occur to me: this is a guy who probably wakes up clean-shaven every morning wearing a perfectly pressed uniform shirt.

'How are you?' I asked him. 'Have you got the kids ready?'

'They're ready,' he said. 'Six of them. I fasted them from zero-six-hundred like you asked.'

That's when I had to deliver the day's first bit of bad news. 'Unfortunately,' I told Dr Pak, 'we've only got four full face masks that will fit the boys. So there will only be four going today.'

Dr Pak didn't complain about the late change, and neither did anyone else. A couple of the kids might have been relieved, or they might have been disappointed. I had no way of knowing which. All I knew was that someone would have to decide which four of the six were still set to go. How'd you like to make that call? As with all the other decisions about which order the kids would go in, it wouldn't be up to the divers who would try to deliver them out. It would be up to Dr Pak, Coach Ekk and the boys themselves.

Together, they would figure it out somehow. I had no idea who my first patient would be.

From the bottom of the hill, I could see that some of the boys had already pulled on the wetsuits that the British divers had brought in over the previous few days. Were they itching to go – or what? I gave Dr Pak a strip of alprazolam tabs that I fetched from the goodie bag. 'You might as well hang on to these,' I said to him. 'I want each kid to take one tablet when I call for him. Don't give it until I say so.'

It was such a relief to have a real medical pro looking after the boys. When Dr Pak said he would take care of something, I had no doubt that he would. 'So go ahead and give the first kid a tablet,' I said. Dr Pak nodded, then headed back up the slippery slope to the boys. Jason was right on his heels.

The first boy was one of the taller ones.

His name was Prachak Sutham, but his friends all called him Note. He'd turned fifteen exactly one week earlier, the eighth day the boys were trapped in the cave. An easygoing eighth-grader at Mae Sai Prasitsart School, the same one attended by Tern, Night, Mick and Dom, Note was known as a bright, quiet boy who tended to do what he was told. He had a two-year-old sister at home and a father who worked in a local auto-repair shop, where Note helped out on weekends. 'When you teach him how to fix something in the garage,' one of the father's co-workers would marvel to CNN, 'he'll learn how to do it after just one go.' Note wasn't just one of the stronger players on the Wild Boars soccer team, he also knew and avidly followed the game. He was an ardent fan of the Thai Premier League's Chiang Rai United. But Jason knew none of that, and neither did I, as the hard-driving British diver began to prepare Note for his risky underwater trip. All we knew was that this boy was the first one, and it was Jason's daunting responsibility to get him out alive.

As the boy stood silently in front of him – lean, squinting in the darkness, black hair swept back and to the right – Jason made sure the wetsuit fitted snugly. He adjusted the diving hood and then the buoyancy device that went over the boy's head like a life jacket on an aeroplane, double-checking the oral inflator and the string that's supposed to dump the air with a single, stiff pull. This device could keep a diver – even an unconscious one, we hoped – neutral in the water, preventing him from floating too high or sinking too low.

While Jason performed each check and manoeuvre, the three Thai Navy SEALs stared intently, trying to learn the pre-dive routine so they might repeat it with future boys. That could speed future rescues, assuming there were any.

Jason wrapped a bungee around Note's chest and a second one around the boy's waist. He wrapped a cable tie around each of the boy's wrists and a second tie through each of those to make a little loop.

'It's to stop water from going into your wetsuit,' Jason told the boy, half in English, half in pantomime. That was true as far as it went. What Jason didn't mention was the other, larger reason for the cable ties: to secure the boy's hands behind his back just before the dive, when the cable ties would be clipped together with a spring-loaded metal carabiner. Some critics in the international media would later howl in outrage at this, declaring that innocent children had been handcuffed like hardened prisoners. That was an ignorant complaint. Securing the boys' hands that way was an important safety measure, protecting their extremities from getting twisted, banged or mangled along the way. It would also ensure that if a boy did wake up unexpectedly, he wouldn't rip off his face mask and drown. For a similar reason, the boys' feet would also be bound before their long dives out. When people panic underwater, even small boys, they can have great strength and be extremely dangerous to both themselves and their rescuers.

We wanted sleek, tight, human packages, gliding through the water as compact as could be.

An 'inert patient package' – that was the expression that Rick coined. I'm all for giving credit where credit is due. And that one needed an acronym, I thought: the SIPP, short for the Stanton Inert Patient Package. Calling them packages or SIPPs was one way we helped dissociate ourselves from the fact that these were indeed living, breathing young human beings whom we could easily be sending to their deaths. Much as we cared about these children, we had a job to do that required technical proficiency and a certain emotional distance. That was always a struggle for me.

As Jason continued with his dive-prep routine at the boys' elevated camp site, I was readying my own makeshift anaesthetic room at the bottom of the slope. I tried to choose the spot carefully. I wanted a flat, stable, water's-edge location where I could lay out what I'd need, have room to work and, just as important, get a small measure of privacy for myself and the boy. I didn't need a cheering section – or a booing mob – weighing in along the way. We could save that for the Wild Boars' next soccer match.

What I settled on was far from ideal. I'd be standing waist-deep in the turbid water at the base of the slope, my drugs balanced precariously on the open pouch I had suspended from the nearby line. I'd have none of the comforts or equipment I was used to in actual hospitals, even the raggedy ones in far-off places I'd worked in over the years. Here, there was no electricity. No decent light other than the one on my caving helmet. No beeping monitors. No high-tech machines. No talented surgeons at my side. No techs or nurses, or so much as a squirt bottle of hand sanitiser or clean strip of gauze. I was in the remotest of locations performing the most rudimentary field medicine under the direst conditions and very much at the mercy of the latest weather report. It was just my young patient, my syringes, my atropine, my ketamine, my wits and me – and some of the best cave divers on the planet.

The world would discover soon enough whether we were any good at this or not.

'We're going to take you down to Dr Harry now,' Jason said, once the boy was finally outfitted and the alprazolam was beginning to take a grip. The anti-anxiety tablet, I hoped, would quell any last-minute jitters. It would also – and I hadn't thought enough about this part – make the kid a little woozy.

As I looked up and saw the groggy boy wobbling down the muddy slope, I did briefly wonder: *Should I have waited for the kid to climb down before I drugged him up?*

Too late now.

Yes, he was a light-footed Thai soccer boy. But he looked almost as clumsy as a middle-aged Australian anaesthetist flopping down all fifteen metres of that 45-degree slope. I hoped he wouldn't fall and land squarely on his doctor before the procedure even began.

17

First Boy

Harry

Ready, steady – *come on down.*

As Note wobbled down the slope in his wetsuit, buoyancy collar and hood, I was waiting not-so-patiently at the bottom of the hill, up to my waist in water. Jason was one step behind him. But I was still holding my hands out, ready to catch the boy in case he lost his footing or came crashing down in the general vicinity of my head.

That wasn't a sign of excess caution. It was an understanding of brain chemistry and gravity. He was drugged with alprazolam, and bodies not locked down tend to tumble towards the centre of the earth.

I was in my wetsuit. I had my glasses on, which I had carefully transported down the front of my wetsuit. I had on my hood and my helmet, which had lights attached. I was still wearing the harness I clip my tanks to, but I'd left the tanks, my mask and my fins over on the beach. Under conditions like these, that's about as undressed as I can be and still be able to work.

Maybe it was the adrenaline of the moment or my relief that we were finally getting started with the job we had come here to do. Or maybe I'd just had time to catch my breath after the long dive in. But I was starting to feel a little better. Not great, but better. I wasn't quite as convinced I was getting the flu.

As the boy reached the bottom, Jason at his side, Pak was only a couple of steps behind. I was already getting myself into position, half in the dirt beside the hill, half in the coffee-coloured water below. We were really going to do this.

I pushed my left knee into the mud and positioned the kid so he was balanced on my right thigh. It was an awkward position, but I needed to lean into the mud to stop myself from sliding any further into the water. Once I got the boy to sit there, I started talking to him.

Babbling, really.

'What's your name?'

'How old are you?'

At the same time, I was patting the boy on the shoulder and steadying him on my knee.

'Good boy, good boy,' I said. 'What position do you play on the soccer team? My name's Harry. I'm a doctor. We're going to get you out of here. Are you ready to go home yet? Or would you prefer to hang out in the cave a little longer?'

Since the boy spoke so little English, roughly equivalent to the amount of Thai I know, I didn't get too many answers during our get-to-know-you interview. He did mention that his name was Note. But the point of all that chatter really wasn't for us to swap biographies. It was for me to calm and distract him. That's one of the things anaesthetists do, along with sending the patients off and making sure they come back alive. We fill the air and ease the nerves. If I distracted young Note well enough, who knew? He might not even notice that I was about to jab a needle into his thigh – and then a second one.

In the operating theatre, I like to have the little ones sitting on their mum's lap. I'll come in close and touch them and start babbling. Say whatever pops into my mind. Just talk rubbish so it all seems routine.

I turned to Pak, inviting him into our little chat. 'Tell him I'm Dr Harry, and I'm a famous soccer player myself.'

Pak shot me a conspiratorial smile and pressed ahead. I could tell everyone was trying to make a bit of a joke of it. It was all gelling. Pak is such an upbeat, optimistic guy, it's hard to feel like there's any danger when he's around, the bloody legendary Thai hero. He was an awesome co-conspirator. He just got it. He was fully on board with the fact that we had to make these kids feel like this was just a normal day at the office for everyone.

Then, without making a big deal of it, I put my left hand on Note's leg and held up the syringe with my right. I blurted out a quick: 'Ready for the injection?'

'Oh, okay,' the boy nodded.

I squeezed a shot of atropine through the thin rubber of his wetsuit and into his leg, feeling each layer of resistance as I went. Rubber. Skin. Muscle. I had done this often enough to stop before I hit bone.

I could see him screw up his eyes a little. There was a bit of a sting. Then I pulled out the needle and rubbed his leg and said in the most compelling tone I had: 'Well done. Good work.'

I leaned over and stuck the syringe into the mud so the needle would be safe for now.

I stared at the boy for a second, trying to gauge how he was. He looked totally fine. He wasn't crying or breathing hard or seeming the least bit jumpy. His attitude was more like, *I've had shots before. That was another shot. It wasn't so bad. I'm brave.*

Then, I pulled out the second syringe, the ketamine.

'There will be a second one,' I said, as matter-of-factly as I could. Again, no alarm. No drama. Routine as could be.

I gave the other leg a quick rub.

'Here comes the ketamine.'

Needle in, no problem, no yelp, no tears.

In addition to a slight facial scrunch-up, I got something else from Note as the ketamine began spreading out from the large muscle at the front of his thigh. He gave me the slightest little thank-you bow.

Which I found totally endearing.

To me, the *wai* is one of the sweetest things about being in Thailand, the ubiquity of that hands-together bow. Thais, male and female, young and old, rich and poor, execute that gesture as a friendly greeting, as an expression of affection, as a note of simple acknowledgement and as a sign of deep respect. Usually accompanied by a slight knee-bend and a pacific smile, that one movement has meanings I cannot even comprehend. A similar move appears elsewhere in South-East Asia and in parts of India, but nowhere is it such a part of life as in Thailand. As the Thais like to point out, in their country even Ronald McDonald clasps his hands in a *wai*.

It's a rich and nuanced tradition, cultural and spiritual both. Thais even bow to visitors from abroad, who are welcome to bow back, no matter how clumsily.

I'd jabbed a needle into each of Note's thighs and, instead of tears, I got a bow in return. What else do you need to know about the gentleness of the Thai people?

It was hard for me to imagine anyone bowing back home. It's not a gesture that travels everywhere well. But Note gave me that little bow as he faded towards unconsciousness, and I have to say I appreciated it.

While the ketamine did its thing, Jason was standing near us at the bottom of the hill, holding a full face mask ready for the boy, waiting for some kind of signal from me that, yes, I had delivered the one-two injections of atropine and ketamine, that Note was adequately anaesthetised and that we could continue preparing the boy for the arduous, multi-hour journey, above and below the water line, that we all hoped would deliver our young friend safe and sound from the cave.

Jason tested the mask a couple more times, holding it up against his own face to make sure it was breathing all right. So far, so good. At the same time, I was holding the fading boy as securely as I could – left hand on the back of his head, right hand supporting his jaw, keeping the airway open until I was sure he was completely unconscious.

Five minutes was all that took.

'Right-o, Jason.'

With that, Jason came to stand in front of Note and me and placed the mask against the boy's placid face, covering everything from just north of his little eyebrows to a spot south of his chin. I held the mask in place while Jason pulled the straps around the back and tightened them.

Jason took extra care making sure the straps were as tight as possible and no part of the diving hood had slipped inside the mask, minimising any risk of leakage. Next step: making sure the kid was still breathing now that the mask was on, which wasn't a given at all.

There's a natural diving reflex I was concerned about, especially with inexperienced divers, even more especially with children: cold things on your face can make you hold your breath. It's a well-known phenomenon. This can last for fifteen or twenty seconds, sometimes even longer. At that point, the person will start gasping for air. So the suspended breathing isn't usually fatal or even all that dangerous. But it's a rocky way to start such a long and dangerous cave dive, and I wanted to keep an eye out for it this time.

Note was breathing fine.

At this point, Jason and I reclined the boy backwards, his feet in the water, his head still out. Jason slid the air cylinder beneath the two bungees, the chest bungee snapping around the cylinder neck, the waist bungee securing the lower part of the tank. He dropped a three- or four-pound weight into the pocket on the front of the buoyancy device. Then, I performed my first pre-dive test, which tested me as much as it tested the boy.

Rolling Note over, I pushed his face into the water and held it there. That felt so wrong to me, just wrong, shoving the face of an unconscious child underwater and holding it there. As a gesture, it was so close to drowning a child. But I needed to see if he was still breathing steadily through the mask even as his mouth and nose were fully submerged. There was a simple way to tell. Were bubbles floating to the surface of the water? Bubbles equal breathing, which equals life.

There were bubbles. I could see them, being exhaled in strong bursts. I stared at them carefully in the harsh, white beam of my helmet light as the bubbles streamed out of the mask, up to the surface of the water and then disappeared. Note was breathing well, and water did not appear to be leaking into the mask. When I lifted his head out of the water, the inside of the mask looked dry.

This, all by itself, was a monumental accomplishment. A sedated child was breathing underwater, completely unconscious, inhaling and exhaling full breaths of air. In the history of scuba, in the history of anaesthesia, in the history of children, I'm not sure this had ever been attempted before, much less achieved.

At this point, Jason went off to collect his own dive gear, which he'd left on the beach across the water at the far side of chamber 9. He suited up for the arduous journey out, a dive that would be like no other ever attempted, accompanied by an unconscious fifteen-year-old. I used the time to do some additional testing. Again, I positioned the boy face down in the water, let him breathe there, then sat him up again, making sure the head straps were tight enough and no water had snuck into the mask. I did that a couple of times. Dry as a bone. I cinched the mask straps up one more time to be sure.

When Jason returned, he took a few minutes to test his own equipment, then helped me with Note's final prep list. Quickly, I glanced up the hill, but no curious little eyes watching, not that I saw. With Note still face down in the water, we pulled his hands behind his back, restraining them with the wrist-tie cable loops and the spring-loaded carabiner. The symbolism of that also seemed terrible to me. However pure our intentions, we were indeed hand-cuffing this child. Then, Jason used another bungee to bind the boy's ankles loosely together. All of it was disquieting but necessary. As we had learned so vividly from our own dives in and out, some of the openings in this cave were ridiculously narrow. Note's trim body had to be as compact and as contained as humanly possible. We couldn't risk him getting snagged on anything along the way.

With that, they were almost ready to go.

Jason had two ways of holding onto young Note in the water and guiding him along. There was a small handle on the back of the boy's buoyancy device that Jason could grip onto, either swimming side by side or gliding along the surface with the boy an easy arm's length below. Jason also clipped a one-metre length of rope to Note's back. If the British diver chose to, he could clip the other end of the rope to his own harness. That way, he wouldn't risk dropping the line and letting the child float away, even if his own hands got busy doing something else. That would be embarrassing, not to mention potentially deadly.

'You ready?' I asked Jason.

He nodded. Jason was always ready.

The drugs had done what they were supposed to. So had Pak. So had I. The boy was fully sedated and all suited up. His mask wasn't leaking. His underwater breathing was strong. Neither Jason nor I had any idea how long any of that would continue to be true. But all the signs said, *Go*.

As Jason waded deeper into the water, with the boy floating beside him, I lingered at the bottom of the hill with Pak just above me. We stood silently there for a moment, knowing exactly how much was at stake here, neither one of us saying a word.

By then, the British diver and the Thai boy were swimming off down the tunnel, only the back of Jason's wetsuit visible from where we were.

That's when I turned to Pak and said: 'Next kid. Next tablet.'

What was I thinking?

I said it without remembering that I was supposed to wait for Jason and his boy to reach chamber 8, where they were going to meet up with Rick, Mikko and Claus and Craig, who would perform a thorough check-up on the boy. Then, Rick would swim back to me with our very first progress report: had boy number one survived the first leg of the high-risk journey? Were we killing these children or saving them? What was working flawlessly? What should we avoid at all cost?

I'm not sure why I was in such a hurry. But with the first boy so painlessly on his way – *not a single tear* – all my instincts told me: get on with boy number two. Maybe it was the efficiency born of twenty years in private practice! Maybe I just didn't like sitting around.

As with the choice of Note, none of the foreign rescuers had any role in deciding who would be next. That was up to Coach Ekk, Dr Pak, the Thai Navy SEALs and, most of all, the boys themselves. They had whatever system they had up on the hill. It was all in their hands.

Number two turned out to be fourteen-year-old Natthawut Thakhamsai – Tern to his friends. Another eighth-grader at Mae Sai Prasitsart School, Tern was listed on the official Wild Boars roster as a defender. But he was even more beloved as the team's unofficial comedian, easily able to make everyone erupt in laughter with his goofy faces, his hilarious jokes and his wicked mimicry. With his twinkly eyes and gap-toothed grin, it was almost impossible not to like Tern, his friends all agreed. And now, if things kept going smoothly, he'd really have something to smile about.

Pak and I were joined at the chamber 9 beach by John Volanthen and Chris Jewell, two of Rick Stanton's other aces. John was up next. It would be his responsibility to ferry young Tern out of the cave. They were a good match. Long before John became a world-class cave diver, he had got his own start in caves as a fourteen-year-old Scout. Now, he'd be taking a fourteen-year-old on his very first cave dive, a trip that just might save the boy's life. Was that a nice circle – or what? But I'd say John was even quieter than usual, the gravity of the situation weighing heavily on him.

With his help and Pak's, I repeated the exact same drill on Tern that Jason and I had performed on Note. Anti-anxiety tablet. Wobbly stumble down the slippery slope to the water. Soothing chit-chat on my knee. Atropine in one leg, ketamine in the other. A five-minute slide into dreamland. Suited up. Faced down. Underwater breathing tests. Tied up like a parcel at Australia Post. And off they swam, John with one hand on the guide rope, one hand on sedated Tern's back handle, down the chamber 9 tunnel towards Craig and the divers I could only assume were waiting in chamber 8. Boy number two was on his way.

By racing ahead prematurely, I hadn't left much room between the first two teams. I certainly didn't want to start the rescue mission with a blind, muddy-water traffic jam. I could only hope that, with a little luck, the second team didn't bang into the first team from behind. And what if Rick was on his way to chamber 9 and crashed into John and Tern in a narrow part of the cave? Now we weren't just talking a rear-ender. We were talking a head-on collision too.

Yes, this was my first official screw-up.

So after feeling like I had a bit of a rhythm going, I was suddenly feeling nervous. Where the hell was Rick? I had already sent two boys into the murky abyss. What horrible fate had befallen them? Maybe in some witch's brew of panic and raw strength, they had already dragged their own rescuers down with them. In the absence of hard information, the mind has an extraordinary capacity for vivid scenarios. Without Rick's report, I had no information at all. The risks were undeniable. Nothing that had happened so far had quelled my profound doubts about the rescue plan, not even the promising launches for the first two boys. With the added burden of knowing I had sent the second boy sooner than I should have, failing to wait for Rick's progress report, I felt alone with my thoughts.

If only I knew what was happening in chamber 8.

18

Chamber 8

Craig

The tiniest vibration – that's all it was at first. I had my fingers on the line, waiting for a sign of movement, and then, yes, the slightest little quiver. Not much. Not yet. No major jerking or yanking around. Just some barely perceptible rope movement alerting me that someone was coming towards us and we'd better get ready for a burst of activity.

How long had Rick and I been waiting in chamber 8? An hour? Longer? Not long but long enough for Harry, Pak and Jason to get the first boy suited up and into the water and long enough for Jason to dive him most of the first leg of the journey out of the cave. It's about a 300-metre dive through the sump from chamber 9 to chamber 8. Figure on twenty minutes for an experienced diver alone, obviously a bit more than that escorting a sedated boy, especially the first one.

I couldn't see anything yet. The water was murky. The helmet lights are never bright enough. Rick and I were on the beach at the edge of the water, peering out towards chamber 9. It would have been nice if Mikko and Claus were there too. So what had happened?

Where were the two European divers who were supposed to help us get the boy across the dry terrain of chamber 8?

Mikko Paasi and Claus Rasmussen were tough, experienced divers. Claus, the Dane with medical and injection experience, had worked with refugees and asylum seekers before moving to Thailand and joining Ben Reymenants's dive business. We knew his talent for languages – he seemed fluent in Thai – would come in handy communicating with the boys. Harry and I had just met Mikko, though we wouldn't soon forget him, not with his shoulder-length dreadlocks, his driven attitude and his weightlifter's physique. A native of Finland, Mikko is the founder of a diving centre on the small Thai island of Koh Tao, where he specialises in ocean and wreck diving. These were not no-show guys.

So what happened to them? They'd either stopped too early, gone really slowly or got sidetracked along the way. Whatever the explanation, it wasn't just the Europeans' extra hands we were hoping to take advantage of once Jason and Note arrived. We were also eager for the sked they were bringing with them.

A sked is a compact rescue stretcher designed for confined spaces, a flat piece of tough plastic that rolls up into the size of a big sleeping-bag. These skeds are amazingly rugged. You can drag them. You can move them through the water fairly easily. You can strap the patient in and transport him across damn near anything. The sked protects against injury. It's easy for a rescuer to use. Just walk in front and pull. It would be perfect, we figured, for delivering sedated boys across what everyone expected would be an especially gnarly dry section of the cave. But since Mikko and Claus hadn't turned up yet, neither had their green sked.

Fairly quickly after the rope began to move, the glow of lights started appearing in the brown sump water between chamber 8 and chamber 9. Dim at first, then gradually brighter. Then, the light got closer – still not a sound – until bubbles began to appear. That's when a diver's helmet popped out of the water. It was Jason.

He stopped right at the point where the beach goes down into the water. He knelt there for a second, organising himself, then flashed a tight smile of recognition at Rick and me and passed the boy up the beach as far as he could push. Jason was in dive gear, so he wouldn't be all that much use on land. Rick and I were just in our wetsuits, much freer to move.

I didn't know which boy it was, his name or background or anything like that – just that it was one of the boys. Over time, I would learn to tell the difference: Is it a big one? Is it a small one? For now, though, I just knew that without the sked, he was going to be heavy, whoever he was. At this point, he was still a patient, someone who needed to be examined, perhaps consoled, maybe sedated again and sent on his way as quickly and efficiently as possible. This was a complex operation, and we were a vital part of it.

As gently as we could, Rick and I pulled his body about halfway onto the beach, his head and chest on the sand, his feet still dangling in the water. We rolled him onto his side, which made it easier to get the cylinder off his chest, then rolled him the rest of the way onto his back, face up. I took his full face mask off, then pulled him the rest of the way out of the water. That's when I got my first good look at his face.

'He's still breathing,' Jason said.

We waited for Jason to say something else, but I guess that was his main focus and his main worry, and Jason was right. The boy was breathing. There was nothing more important than that. I put my fingers loosely up to the boy's mouth. The breath felt steady and strong. Then, I continued with what I would call a rudimentary veterinary field examination.

I pulled his lip up and looked at the colour of his gums to make sure they were nice and pink – not blue.

They were pink.

I checked the capillary refill time, pressing on the gum until it turned white. Then, I released my finger. The gum should turn pink again in one second, definitely no longer than two. That tells us how well the patient's blood is flowing to the peripheral parts of his body. The white disappeared fast. From that I knew his heart was beating well and his blood flow was strong.

I felt inside his mouth to see if he was warm. His temperature was fine, which I expected. He hadn't been in the water all that long, including the time that Harry and Jason were gearing him up. While I was focused on the boy's mouth, I also made sure he hadn't vomited and that he didn't have a lot of saliva coming out. Things seemed fairly dry in there. None of this was a hospital-level examination. In fact, doctors reading this are probably shaking their heads, aghast. But I had none of the equipment or other conditions for anything more. Taken together, it was a good basic once-over, and he was coming through fine. All along, I was looking for signs that the boy might be waking from his anaesthetic slumber. Were his hands moving? Were his feet? I checked his palpebral reflex, tapping in the corner of his eye and seeing if the eyelid moved. That's a very early sign of lightening anaesthetic. His eyelid did twitch vigorously as I tapped there.

He wasn't wide awake. Not even close. But his sleep was definitely lighter than was ideal. 'We need to top him up,' I said to Rick, who readily agreed.

I reached into my kit and removed one of the syringes so I could administer a half-dose of ketamine, a drug I'd given to countless dogs and other animals over the years. Though Note would be my first drowsy boy, I felt fully prepared. As Harry pointed out, I'd probably given a lot more ketamine than he had. It's a drug that's used far less routinely with humans than with animals. I know how they respond to it. I know what they look like when they're waking up. I can tell how much more is needed. All those responses, I reasoned, should be similar with these boys, who weren't any larger than some of the big dogs I had treated and definitely smaller than the horses and kangaroos. I would never claim to have anywhere near the expertise that Harry has as an anaesthetic specialist, far from it. But generally speaking, in veterinary surgery, one person is both the surgeon and the anaesthetist. So I'd sedated patients thousands of times.

I poked the needle through the thin wetsuit and into the boy's thigh. I gave the syringe a gentle squeeze. Soon, I could see his sleep deepen. That part was easy. What came next was hard.

Jason was still in most of his dive gear. So he wasn't much good to us as a physical hauler on land. Claus, Mikko and their sked still hadn't arrived. That left Rick and me to lug the clumsy weight of a sleeping boy across the long dry section of chamber 8.

We grabbed him under his arms while also supporting his head, Rick on the left, me on the right, our grips wrapped from armpit to shoulder. His feet more or less dragged behind. It wasn't the smoothest form of locomotion or the easiest for us to pull off. But each step got us one step closer to the water at the other side of the chamber, where Jason could resume the long dive out.

We didn't mind dragging the boy's feet on the sandy beach or in the shallow water along the way. That was okay. But when we got to the rocky section further along, then we had to carry him. For that stretch, Rick and I changed positions. I held the boy's ankles.

Rick had the underarm grip. That was actually difficult. Note wasn't particularly big or heavy. But you know how hard and clumsy a manoeuvre like that can be if you've ever tried to carry a limp person any distance at all.

Jason didn't waste any time. He was busy too. He moved all his own gear across the dry part of the chamber and then walked back and got the kid's cylinder, mask and vest. The gear was easy enough for Jason to carry, even half-outfitted as he was.

There was a bit of a duck we had to get through. It wasn't long at all, only a couple of yards. There was water to wade across. At one stage, it was chest-deep. Then it was neck deep. But we could always touch the bottom, and we held firmly onto Note, keeping his head above water. This was definitely a walk, not a dive, and we just kept plodding forwards. The speed broke no records, but our progress was steady enough. There was another duck at the far end, the demarcation between chamber 8 and chamber 7. Later in the rescue, as that water dropped, the two chambers would become a single chamber with no sump and no duck between them, just an imaginary line. But for now, we still had to duck through.

Jason had all the dive gear waiting there for us, his and Note's both. When we arrived, he was getting himself ready to climb back into the water.

I asked Jason how he was doing.

'The diving's okay,' he said. 'But I'm not feeling right in the water. There might be something wrong with the air we're breathing.'

First, Harry. Now, Jason. And come to think of it, I wasn't feeling so hot myself.

It hadn't really occurred to me before. But I'd had a headache on the dive in, which is rare for me. None of us had been drinking the night before, and I was well hydrated. So there was no obvious explanation other than the air in the tanks. Rick piped up and said the air smelled bad to him. When we got out of the cave, we agreed, we would have to check what was going on with the compressor that was being used to fill the tanks. But there was nothing to do about it now. We would just have to proceed, bad air or not. Luckily, the boys were breathing 80 per cent oxygen with only a small amount of air in their cylinders. So they shouldn't be affected.

Rick and I began assembling the boy's equipment and getting him shipshape to dive again. We were definitely learning our procedures on this first transfer and check-up exercise, but I had every confidence we'd keep getting better as more boys came through and we got to keep practising our moves.

I checked the boy's sedation level one last time. He seemed fully out to me. We wished him luck and wished Jason luck and sent them on their way.

Rick knew that Harry was waiting in chamber 9 to hear his early report – or, as it would turn out, *not* waiting but still needing to hear it. Rick was also supposed to dive boy number four out of the cave. But with still no sign of Mikko and Claus, he didn't want to leave me alone in chamber 8. Would I need him to help carry the next boy across? But was Harry waiting for Rick before sending another boy through?

We didn't have to wait long to find out.

The rope began moving again. The lights appeared in the water. It was quicker than either of us expected, but here was boy number two and his able British dive escort, John Volanthen.

'His name is Tern,' John said to Rick and me after emerging from the water. 'Have a look, but he seems to be doing okay.'

I was happy to hear that. I was also happy to notice that the second boy seemed a little smaller – and a little lighter, I hoped – than the first one. Luckily, things were going well so far. If something had gone horribly wrong and Rick had been helping me and not delivering word to Harry and then Harry had sent along the next boy, we would have had another one arriving while still trying to deal with the first one. Who knows what that would have meant? Luckily, that didn't happen – not yet.

We pulled young Tern out of the water and stripped off the heavy parts of his gear. John took off some of his own. Like Jason before him, he would lug the boy's equipment and then his own to the far side of the chamber.

I could tell right away that Tern would also need a ketamine top-up. His vitals all looked solid – breathing, temperature, blood flow. But he was definitely twitchy in his sedation. This was already becoming a pattern. One dose was not going to be enough, not for a nine-chamber dive as long and complex as this one. I gave Tern the shot before Rick and I got the best grips we could and began carrying him. Across the sand. Just about to the rocky section. Then, without a word of warning, Claus and Mikko appeared.

I didn't get a straight story about exactly what had delayed them. Apparently, they had thought they were supposed to be at a different location. Never having dived this far into the cave, they weren't exactly sure of the layout. They wanted to hear how things had been going and were eager to be helpful. But I noticed something right away.

'Where's the sked?' I asked Claus and Mikko.

The stretcher, for some reason, was back at the near side of chamber 7.

'Well, go and get it,' I snapped. 'We need it.'

Rick was getting eager to head back and out to chamber 9. He needed to report to Harry. He needed to get his own boy. But he stayed with me and with Tern while Claus and Mikko went off to fetch the stretcher. When they got back, we had carried Tern most of the way across the chamber anyway.

Despite the rocky start, Mikko and Claus would prove to be hugely valuable partners as the mission rolled on. Claus could handle just about anything. Mikko was strong as a bull, able to drag that sked across any imaginable terrain, no problem at all, with minimal assistance from anyone. Half the time I was running just to keep up with him.

19

Night Moves

Harry

'It's all good, Harry,' Rick said once he'd climbed out of the water and sat next to me on the little beach at chamber 9.

You can imagine how relieved I was to hear that.

'The first two kids have come through,' Rick went on. 'They seem fine. They're breathing. They're asleep. Good work. Carry on.'

I had to take a moment to absorb that. Not knowing had caused more anxiety than I had realised. I let out a huge sigh when I heard Rick's news. My pounding heart needed time to slow down. Sending these boys off in decent shape was nice. Hearing that they'd made it through their first check-up in decent shape was way, way better. I took a moment just to bask in that. This entire rescue mission, I was coming to see, would ultimately become a series of slowly revealed unknowns. Well, two of those unknowns had now been revealed. In the scheme of things, this might sound like a small accomplishment. Believe me, hearing those words from Rick was huge.

I was also feeling close to normal now, and I was more certain about why I'd felt so crappy on my way into the cave. It had to be bad gas in my cylinder. There was really no other explanation for it. I'd felt fine before I went into the water. I hadn't eaten anything risky. And I was feeling much better now. Even accounting for the pressure and the adrenaline of our day so far, what could it be but the gas? Once I quit breathing from the tank and was sucking in cave air, I felt all right. We would have to check on the gas-filling operations at the end of the day and try to ensure this didn't happen again. Killing the whole rescue team, no matter how many kids survived our risky recipe, would not be a good start to proceedings.

It was much too soon to get cocky. We still had eleven rescues to go. But it's fair to say I liked the way this was going. We were on a little roll.

The boys were easily sedated. The divers were getting them out, at least a few hundred metres into the next chamber. Rick mentioned an issue in chamber 8 – something about Claus and Mikko and a missing stretcher – but Rick said everyone was now good to go. His report could hardly have been more encouraging, and now he was talking next steps with Pak and me in chamber 9, as was Chris Jewell. Chris would be ferrying boy number three, once the ketamine and I did our thing.

I still had no idea how the first boys were faring once they moved past Craig and Rick in chamber 8. Knowing the cave as I was beginning to, I was fully aware of the many perils that lay ahead from there. The boys could awaken in an underwater section where giving a top-up would be nigh-impossible. In tight areas with no visibility, they faced the constant danger of banging their heads against the rock, even though the divers tried to minimise that risk and protect the boys' heads against the stalactites and unpredictable ceiling drops – going so far as allowing their own heads to take a bit of a beating. But what if a boy's torso got jammed in one of the many tiny openings? What if the passage was too narrow for him, his escort and their tanks? What if the boy's mask became dislodged? There are many ways to drown inside a flooded cave. But I couldn't distract myself with a thousand scenarios. I had to stay focused on my responsibilities, anaesthetising number three and then number four and getting them on their way, with adequate space between them this time.

I had learned that lesson, right?

The third boy was Pipat Bodhi. His friends all called him Nick. He'd had his fifteenth birthday the day before the Wild Boars went into the cave. A student at Ban San Sai School, he wasn't even a member of the team. But he'd tagged along to practice that day with his friend, goalie Ekkarat 'Biw' Wongsookchan. When the boys headed off to the cave after practice, Nick happily came too. A bright boy who sometimes struck new acquaintances as stiff and serious, his extroverted, witty side would always come out, as would his passion for Mookata Thai barbecue, as soon as he felt comfortable, people who knew him well explained.

I didn't get to see any of that. By the time Pak gave the boy the anti-anxiety tablet and Chris got him suited up and the two of them pointed him down the slope, Nick wasn't saying much of anything. He was gentle and utterly compliant when he settled on my knee. We engaged in the usual blather. I gave him the usual shots. He responded with the quiet bravery I was getting used to. Barely any wincing at all.

Rick stood by, seeing for the first time how we did things in the farthest chamber. Chris pulled on the rest of his own gear and swam back to where I sat with an anaesthetised Nick. Chris Jewell was exactly the sort of bloke I wanted on this mission. At thirty-five, he was the youngest of the Brits. A key member of the Cave Diving Group of Britain and Northern Ireland, he served as the group's main liaison with the British Cave Rescue Council. Chris was the one who'd organised the 2013 diving expedition to Mexico's Huautla cave that was the deepest so far discovered in the Western Hemisphere. Young, smart and strong, Chris seemed like exactly the right man for this rescue.

And off they went, Chris and Nick, towards chamber 8 and, we could only hope, towards the friends and family and worldwide audience that had been so desperately cheering for the boys' safe release from the cave. Another one on his way to freedom.

I gave the pair what I believed was plenty of lead time before moving on to the fourth boy, the last of the day, the one Rick Stanton was going to ferry out, Pheeraphat Sompiengjai. With Rick in the water, I had no doubt the boy would be in excellent hands. Known to his friends and family as Night, young Pheeraphat was another June birthday. Since he turned sixteen the day the group went missing, 23 June, he was the oldest player on the soccer team. A student at Mae Sai Prasitsart and a Wild Boars right-winger, Night was blamed by some people for the fact that the children got stuck in Tham Luang cave. That wasn't fair. While it was true that the boys went to the cave in part to celebrate Night's birthday, most of them, like many local children around Mae Sai, had been inside the cave plenty of times. They were happy to have any excuse.

Night's sister was born during the Water Festival. So their father started calling her Nam, water in Thai. Pheeraphat was born after dark. So he became Night. Night was especially close to his parents. Fifteen days earlier, Night's mother, Supaluk, had urged him to hurry home from practice. She had a SpongeBob SquarePants cake waiting for him. Now, Night's mother and father, joined by other relatives, were spending every night sleeping at the cave site.

When Night came down the slope, I recognised that he was one of the boys who seemed to have some chest congestion. I could hear it in his breathing. When I began to talk with him, there was a raspy tone in his voice. He didn't sound seriously ill to me, but there was definitely something going on.

The send-off was normal enough. We followed the same drill we had with the first three boys. Despite or perhaps because of whatever infection he was fighting, Night faded soon after he got the ketamine, perhaps a little more quickly than the other boys. Enough to make me nervous I had given him too much. But each kid would be different. That was to be expected. That's what I told myself, anyway. Rick and I packaged him up according to the recipe. Then, Rick swam off with Night, back towards Mikko, Claus and Craig in chamber 8.

Rick and Night hadn't even made it out of the chamber 9 canal when Rick turned around and called out to me.

'Harry,' he yelled, 'this kid is really not breathing much.'

Rick knew the difference. He'd worked with Craig on the first two boys, whose breathing was perfectly robust. This was different. Rick's alarm was concerning to me. But the truth is, there wasn't much either of us could do about it, much as we would like to – not in the middle of the water.

'Just go, mate,' I yelled back. 'I'm sorry. If you bring him back here, what am I going to do? Just go and get through.'

I knew we had some science on our side. With 80 per cent oxygen in the tank, the boy should need only the three breaths a minute that Rick was counting. That's not ideal, but that rate of breathing will sustain life. He'll be okay. As long as his airway is open and he's getting those three proper breaths of 80 per cent oxygen, he'll be fine.

Rick swam on.

I threw on my dive gear as quickly as I could. Despite all the cheery self-talk – *three breaths a minute, 80 per cent oxygen, nothing to worry about* – I was seriously worried. The day had got off to such a promising start. Now *this*? I figured I'd better follow Rick and the slow-breathing boy. 'I'll see you guys tomorrow,' I called out to Pak, again feeling bad that maybe I wouldn't be back at all. With the constant threat of rain, there was no way to know. But I didn't delay or turn back or do anything that would slow me down. I stepped into the water, grabbed hold of the guide rope and moved towards chamber 8 as quickly as my arm pulls and fin kicks could safely carry me.

Now, it was my turn to follow the route the divers and boys were on. The water was worse than I remembered from the morning.

As I inched along the line, the visibility was absolute zero. That's how much silt had been kicked up in the water by the divers and the four human packages they were delivering out of the cave. I didn't even bother keeping my eyes open. I couldn't see anything anyway. I just moved through the murky water – slow and steady – making sure not to drop the line.

Travelling so methodically, I wasn't sure exactly how long it would take to reach chamber 8. Pull, advance, pull, advance, see nothing. It's hard to calculate distance when that's all you have in your head. There was a line trap on the right where the rope pulled tight into an unpassable crevice. It had to be negotiated. There was a flattener where my chest and belly barely scraped through, made slightly easier by the cave's soft clay floor. Then, all of a sudden, I felt something with my right hand, something I didn't recognise.

What was that?

It felt rubbery and cold, and it was down in the mud at the floor of the cave. If I had been diving in the ocean, I'd have thought it was a fish. But that made no sense here. Whatever I touched wasn't wiggling, and there weren't any fish that I knew of in Tham Luang cave.

It took another second before it hit me. *That's a foot, a small, human foot.* It didn't seem to be moving at all.

I still couldn't see anything in the water, but after another second or so, I was able to unwind the obvious: there was a boy attached to the foot, and Rick was attached to the boy.

As if Rick didn't have enough to deal with already: the zero visibility. His kid's chest infection. The exhaustion all of us felt at the end of the day. Now, I was rear-ending him. Then my head popped above the surface just in time to see Rick pulling the boy out of the water and onto the sand. By now, only the boy's legs were submerged.

I yanked my helmet and mask off and spat out my mouthpiece, just as Craig appeared as well. Both of them looked genuinely worried.

'Is everything okay?' I asked.

'I don't think so,' Rick said, glancing down at the boy. 'He's not right. The breathing – I'm not happy with that at all.'

I quickly pulled off the rest of my gear.

'Let's pull him right up on the sand,' I said.

My heart was pumping hard now. This felt very serious to me. As far as I knew, the first boys were out without major incident. At least, they were safely on their way. Was boy number four going to be our moment of truth?

Once Night was fully on the sand, Craig and I rolled him onto his right side. He felt cold. Too cold. He didn't seem to be breathing at all.

I lay on the sand behind him. At first, I wasn't eager to remove his full face mask or cylinder. Whatever benefits he was getting from the 80 per cent oxygen, why disrupt the flow? But I needed to get his breathing going again. When I did slide off the mask, his lips looked blue. My first thought was that he might have been over-dosed with anaesthetic or become hypothermic. I had seen reactions like this before when anaesthetised children had a chest infection. They would often behave badly. They'd hold their breath. They'd get something called laryngeal spasm. Their airways were irritable. It's not their fault. But little buggers with chest infections often play up under anaesthetic. I reached around and lifted Night's chin then slipped my fingers into the front of his mouth, pulling his jaw forwards. That's a standard anaesthetic manoeuvre, a good way to ensure a patient's airway is open and to feel how strong the breath-ing is. Holding my hand in front of his mouth like that, I waited to feel the boy's warm breath on my palm.

I was totally still, instinctively holding my own breath, eager for the slightest indication. I might have felt a little something but not enough to convince myself that he was exhaling anything. If I'd have held a mirror up, I don't think it would have fogged at all.

Then, I placed my hand against the boy's belly, which is another way of checking for respiratory effort. I felt some movement, but again it wasn't remotely regular or strong. A short, occasional breath – that's all I could feel. This kid was really struggling. That much I knew.

I stared at his face. His skin had a blueish tint. Was he blue because he wasn't breathing or blue because he was cold? I couldn't tell. I thought about it for another few seconds, but I couldn't get the notion out of my head. *He's definitely not breathing enough. I'm going to have to roll him over for mouth-to-mouth resuscitation.*

I was just about to do that when his breathing picked up.

Stronger. Steadier. Enough that I could feel his belly moving in and out.

Whew!

I can't tell you how relieved I was to feel that. I reached up to confirm it. And yes, I could now feel warm breath above the boy's chin.

I have never in all my years as a doctor been so excited to feel a burst of hot air. Breath is proof of life, and young Night was breathing.

An experience like that is unsettling in a proper operating theatre. It was positively harrowing on the sands of chamber 8 in Tham Luang cave.

'Okay,' I said to Rick and Craig, as Mikko and Claus looked on. 'I think we're all right now. Let's get him on the stretcher and get him out of here.'

Night's breathing stayed strong, which I was profoundly grateful for. But as Mikko and Claus went off to get the stretcher, another issue developed. The boy, I could tell, was clearly starting to rouse. He was breathing harder and writhing noticeably. He was struggling with his arms behind his back, pulling at the binding around his wrists.

This I knew how to deal with. I knew what he needed. He needed another shot of ketamine. Since I was there, I didn't have to count on anyone else to administer it. I reached into my kit. I removed a syringe. I gave him a booster shot in the thigh.

Keeping the balance right was key, I knew. I didn't want to under-anaesthetise him or he'd surely wake up again in the next chamber or the one after that. I didn't want to over-anaesthetise him and put him out for too long. I definitely did not want another episode like the one we'd just had. All my dose levels so far were guesswork, and this one would be guesswork, too.

There was just so much we didn't know.

I still didn't know about the condition of Note, Tern and Nick – or Night, for that matter. All I knew was that Craig reported that they were alive and seemed fine when they left chamber 8. We knew nothing that happened after that. The most perilous part of the entire cave was the passage from chamber 4 to chamber 3, just past where the ex-Navy SEAL had died and even the most experienced cave divers struggled. We had no idea what our SIPPs might have confronted there.

20

Day's End

Harry

Diving without a sedated child is definitely easier than diving with one.

So Craig and I made better time than any of the four boy-and-diver teams who had left before us, even though their head-starts kept them comfortably in front. No more traffic jams today. We made it through the tricky passage out of chamber 4 and were swimming smoothly into chamber 3, what the Thai Navy SEALs called their forward operating base and what I thought of as our big-box equipment warehouse. I was just lifting my head out of the water at the edge of the chamber 3 beach, when one of the American pararescue guys leaned down, slapped my helmet and said:

'Four out of four, doc.'

At first, I couldn't really process that. There was so much emotion swirling inside me, I jumped straight to the worst possible interpretation. I assumed he meant four out of four had died.

These pararescuers were just awesome. They exuded a sense, whatever was happening around them, that they were completely in charge and could handle anything. He could tell from the look on my face, I suppose, that I wasn't responding appropriately and that I might be having trouble grasping what he had just said to me.

'It's all good,' he emphasised. 'They're all in the hospital. Everyone is okay.'

What a relief that was! I gave it a few seconds to sink in. But even so, the moment felt otherworldly to me. Like we weren't really the ones who had done it. Or that whatever had happened with today's boys might be a weird fluke and tomorrow all of them would die. I was surprised and elated and relieved, but at the same time I wasn't certain that any of this was actually happening for real.

As I pulled myself out of the water and glanced around chamber 3, I could see many people standing there. The British divers were waiting for us, having handed off their boys to the bucket-brigade of Americans, Chinese and Thai medics who delivered them to the field hospital outside the entrance to the cave. So were the Euro divers. The Thai SEALs too. No one seemed in a hurry to go anywhere. We traded a few quick recollections with the Brits and the Euro divers, recalling some of the day's high and low points. The first boy's wobbly trip down the hill. The ever-present risk of traffic jams. The sked that had turned up late to chamber 8. Where had it got to? Rick's delayed report. Night's laboured breathing. Especially Night's laboured breathing. I could still feel the panic that had swept over me until his steady breathing resumed.

No one had any detailed updates on the boys yet. But word was already beginning to trickle in from the field hospital, where the kids were said to be waking up and even talking. I wasn't clear on whether that was one kid or some kids or all of them. I couldn't imagine that Night was bright-eyed yet. And all of it was hearsay at this point. But no one was hearing anything alarming or negative.

We had to keep moving. We couldn't wait in chamber 3 all night.

Craig and I made our way out of the cave and went directly to the Australian Federal Police compound, primarily to sit down, relax a little and catch our breath. We'd been in the cave since ten in the morning. It was now well past eight. I wouldn't say Craig and I were especially talkative. Mainly, we were eager to hear more. But even after another hour, no one seemed to have any real details on the condition of the boys. That made me worry just a little. Was there something we should know?

We trudged up to the British bunker to check in on Rick and his boys. They'd had a long day too. I was eager for their impressions after they'd had time to reassemble and compare notes. If I knew Rick, he'd already be thinking about how we could improve tomorrow. These guys are all about learning from experience, a trait I try to share.

Any early lessons?

It turned out there was a whole lot more to discuss than I had realised. Yes, we'd got the first four out. Yes, they seemed to be doing okay. But as we started to talk, it became quickly apparent that we still had big room for improvement as we proceeded to rescue the next nine Wild Boars.

Craig jumped right in. 'What was the problem with the air in the tanks?' he asked. 'It affected Harry, Rick, Jason and me, probably others too. Nobody felt right. We need clean air tomorrow.'

It sounded like a reasonable request. Far better not to poison the divers!

We all suspected the compressor that had been used to fill the tanks, but Claus was the one who confirmed the issue with the

Thai sailors in charge. 'I went down and talked to the compressor guys to make sure they were changing the filters,' he said. 'I did it in the most correct way I could, asking clarifying questions and giving them ideas about filter run times without saying anything is wrong or anyone is at fault.'

Very deft. Claus had been in Thailand long enough to learn the power of a smile and a thank-you. 'At their naval base, these guys were used to filling only a few tanks at a time,' he said. 'They had never tried anything on this scale.' Apparently, the sailors had run out of filters and so had stopped changing them. It was likely we had all received a dose of hydrocarbons, which gave us those flu-like symptoms. 'They had also managed to fry four boosters including our little portable unit by running too much and too fast,' Claus said. He and one of his diving mates helped the sailors set up a replacement compressor. 'Hopefully, it will last until we're done here.'

Much better.

Some of the issues were relatively small. Someone had noticed that when the first four boys came out of the cave, the tops of their toes were scraped and bloody. Once that was mentioned, it made perfect sense. Unlike the divers who wore wetsuit booties, the boys had nothing on their feet. This was fine as long as they were buoyant in the water. But when the tops of their feet dragged across the sand, silt, pebbles and rocks on the floor of the cave, their toes were getting all banged up. We agreed that, going forwards, the boys would get booties too. This wasn't a life-or-death issue, but no one likes bloody toes. It was just something we hadn't thought about.

A bigger deal was the boys' names, and this was my fault. We could have given them hospital wristbands. There was some talk about that before we went in. With a waterproof pen, I could have written the boys' names in fat capital letters on their arms.

NOTE. NIGHT. That way, when they arrived unconscious at the field hospital, the doctors and nurses would have known who they were. From what we had heard, it wasn't until the boys got to Chiangrai Prachanukroh Hospital that they were identified from photos.

As they'd been waiting outside the cave, the Thai medical personnel team had diligently assembled the boys' medical records, including such worth-knowing details as what drugs each was allergic to. This would have given the trauma team a quick head start on whatever emergency treatments were required. Instead, they had to waste valuable minutes finding people – not the boys' family members – and asking, 'You *sure* this is Note?'

The Thai government preferred not to formally release the names of the boys who'd left the cave until all of them were out.

'We'll find some hospital bands for tomorrow,' I promised.

There was also the subject of the wetsuits. This wasn't so much an issue of health or of danger but of limited supply. As soon as the first boys arrived unconscious at the field hospital, the critical-care team did what they were trained to. They tried to cut the wetsuits off. That's a routine trauma-medical practice. The first thing you do when patients arrive is cut their clothes off. Do you know how awkward it is to get a sleeping patient out of a wetsuit? Very. The nurses went right for the shears.

'Hold on a second,' someone said as they stopped the nurses. 'We need those wetsuits. You can't slice them to pieces.'

Just another one of the details none of us had thought of. Chalk it up to lessons learned.

There was other stuff to keep an eye on. John asked about the weather. John always asked about the weather. He was right to. One crack of thunder could change everything. Everyone agreed we could use more divers. 'They're coming,' Rick said. Then there was the overall flow.

What had we learned by the end of day one, now that we'd got four boys out in the course of a single, long session of sedation and diving? 'So if we do four again tomorrow,' Rick said, 'that will leave five for the third day. Unless we added a fourth day, which I don't think anyone is in favour of. Maybe the coach would like to wait and come out with the Navy SEALs after all the boys are done. Then we could do four, four and four. He's an adult. You think he could dive out with the SEALs – dive out normally, I mean?'

I wasn't sure about that.

'I can ask,' I said. 'I'll have Pak discuss it with him.'

That was about as far as we got when Rick and I were called into a meeting. The Thai medical people wanted to speak with us. With me, especially.

In another squat building with a long folding table, half a dozen sombre-looking men sat on plastic chairs. I got the distinct impression that I wasn't being summoned to receive an award.

'What happened?' the man at the head of the table asked me in English. 'With the fourth boy.'

Night, the fourth boy, was still deeply anaesthetised, the man said. It wasn't clear when the boy would be fully awake. 'You must change the doses,' I was told in no uncertain terms.

'Well,' I said, stalling a moment. 'Let's think about that.'

I wasn't at all sure that lightening the ketamine dose was a good idea. We'd had four successes out of four attempts, hadn't we? As far as I knew, all four of the boys had come out of the cave alive. Given the dim expectations we had started the day with, given all our deep concerns about diving sedated children out of a flooded cave, truthfully I was expecting *high-fives* from the Thai officials – or at least some gentle *good onyas* – not a stern interrogation. Night would wake up eventually. I did not want to mess with the recipe.

So I said no. 'We'll stick with what we're doing.'

I had no idea what reaction that might provoke. This was their country and their cave. These were their children. Ultimately, the Thai government and the Thai medical officials held all the cards. We were invited guests here, outside volunteers. But they let me have my way. I'm not sure if that was because they bought my don't-mess-with-success argument. Or maybe they just liked having me out on a limb alone. That way, at the very earliest catastrophe, I'd be the perfect target for blame.

By the end of the briefing, it wasn't feeling nearly as much like an inquisition as it had at the start. The Thais seemed increasingly persuaded that the early signs were encouraging and things might actually be working out here. It was getting late, after eleven by then. I was completely exhausted. Most of the officials seemed to be as well.

When we got back to the hotel, I said goodnight to Craig and called Fiona while I got ready for bed. She'd been glued to the telly back in Adelaide as various relatives, friends and neighbours kept popping in. She seemed deeply relieved at how things were going at the cave in Thailand. Everything had gone pretty well, I told her. But I said I was still terrified.

'It could all be a weird fluke,' I said of the day's four successful rescues. 'We could easily kill the next four boys. I have this fear that people will start dying on day two.'

Fiona was used to me talking like that. I think she considered it melodramatic. She exuded her usual calm and confidence, whether that was justified or not. I went even further in my mind when we got off the phone. *Our plan is rubbish. Sedating these children is a reckless idea. It could all go to shit on day two.*

I'm not sure if it was Fiona's level-headedness. Maybe I just needed some sleep. I fell asleep immediately. And somehow by Monday morning I had punched my way through most of the doubt. 'At least we got four out,' I told Craig at breakfast. 'That's four more than anyone expected, more than *we* expected.' I wouldn't say I was feeling super-optimistic about the day ahead. But I thought more successes were at least possible, and I was fully convinced that we were the guys to do it.

'So,' I said to Michael Costa as we rode in the DFAT van back to the cave. 'We've got diplomatic immunity now, I suppose.'

'You do,' Michael said.

'I've never had that before. What do you think we could get away with?'

Michael gave me another one of his stricken looks. *Oh*, I thought, *this is going to be fun.*

'Littering?' I asked. 'Would you be able to look after us if we were caught littering?'

'No worries. You'd be fine with that.'

'Okay,' I pressed on. 'What about stealing that Humvee over there?' There was a Humvee parked nearby, a shiny dark-green under the splattered mud.

'I don't think that's a good idea,' he said. He hadn't quite worked us out yet, but he seemed genuinely worried that we would actually steal this car.

Then we probably took it a bit far.

'Any crimes against humanity? Maybe we could . . .?'

He looked thoroughly stricken at that. 'Oh, please,' he begged. 'Don't say that. The government takes that very seriously.'

'All right,' I relented. 'I was teasing about *that*. But we wouldn't mind that Humvee.'

And we never let that go for the rest of the trip.

'We need our own dive vehicle,' Craig kept saying. 'That Humvee is really the only thing that will be satisfactory.'

The ongoing back and forth left him seriously perplexed. But we never backed off the talk of an exciting Humvee heist, and that meant Michael couldn't either. From that point forward, we got daily updates.

'I was looking into the car thing,' he said. 'It's going to be really difficult.'

The rest of the time we were in Thailand, Michael looked nervous whenever we drove past the Humvee.

21

Getting Good

Harry

We were back in the water with a story to tell, and I couldn't wait
to tell it.

As soon as I arrived in chamber 9 for the second day of the rescue,
I told Pak I wanted to talk to the boys. He led me up the slippery
slope again. They all gathered around me on the ledge, the boys, the
coach, the SEALs and Pak. All I could feel were their eyes.

'I have some good news for you,' I said to the children as Pak
translated and everyone else just stared. 'It's about your friends. They
are having a wonderful time in the hospital. They are sleeping in
beds with clean sheets. They are enjoying warm showers. They are
eating their favourite foods.'

The boys started rustling. I could see the smiles breaking out.

'A lot of ice cream,' I said. 'They are all eating ice cream. They
are happy and smiling and talking and laughing and playing
video games.'

Ice cream? Video games? Okay, I might have embellished some
of that. But all of it *could* have been true. And I thought my upbeat

assessment would help to ease the boys' lingering concerns – and might even quiet my own anxieties. I didn't say anything about Night's laboured breathing or my own dark thoughts before bed.

The kids were smiling and upbeat from that point on. If any of them had any doubt, it wasn't being expressed now. All of them seemed ready to give our plan a try. They were keen as mustard, including the coach. And I would soon have fresh reason for confidence too.

On Sunday, the first rescue day, it took about three hours for the divers to bring each boy out. On Monday, we would manage to reduce that to two hours. (By Tuesday, we'd trim it even further, to ninety minutes per boy.) The teamwork got smoother. The journey was that much more familiar to everyone. The divers all knew exactly where they had to be at what time and were getting increasingly practised at what they had to do.

And the Thai officials were starting to relax. For the first time, Governor Narongsak Osottanakorn skipped holding a morning planning meeting. But I still couldn't relax. I was still feeling like I was one injection away from killing a fourteen-year-old, and there were other bumps we had to overcome. This was still a big operation with countless moving parts. When Danish diver Ivan Karadzic showed up at the cave that morning, he did not look well. His complexion was pale. His hands were clammy.

'I'm good to go,' Ivan insisted. He had come to help, and he intended to. Over his protests, a couple of the other divers walked Ivan to the field hospital, where the nurses knew the flu when they saw it. They slapped an IV in his arm and told Ivan he wasn't diving anywhere. That required some last-minute shifting around. Thankfully, Jim Warny, a 35-year-old Belgian diver (and Lufthansa electrician) now living in County Clare, Ireland, had arrived in

Thailand the day before in response to Rick's call. Connor Roe had arrived with Jim. Connor, twenty-six, is a lance corporal in the British Army originally from Somerset, with a permanent smile plastered across his face. The last to arrive was Josh Bratchley, twenty-seven and a meteorologist with the Met Office forecasting service. He's based on the Isle of Anglesey off the north coast of Wales. These were talented younger divers, the United Kingdom's and Ireland's next generation of cave-diving stars, happy to jump on a plane at a moment's notice – and genuinely helpful once they arrived. By midday Monday, with Ivan still in the medical tent too ill to dive to his spot in chamber 6, the three fresh arrivals were stationed at strategic points inside the cave to keep things moving and help with the top-ups as needed. Jim took Ivan's spot in chamber 6. Josh and Connor manned chamber 5. Despite the personnel changes, our one-diver-one-boy system and our deep-sedation strategy didn't change at all. The system had worked well enough on the previous day, and we didn't see any reason to trash it. The tweaks we'd made in the Sunday night meeting would only make it better, right? I could only hope that the Thai medical people, who rightly started out so sceptical, were finally beginning to relax.

Once back in the cave, I was now growing more confident with every injection of ketamine. I was getting more comfortable with the precise doses I delivered, factoring in each kid's weight, appearance and my own clinical gestalt about how much each one could handle. Either this anaesthesia idea was more brilliant than any of us ever imagined or I was beginning to believe my own propaganda.

As Monday got busy, the three Thai Navy SEALs in chamber 9 were taking on a larger role, helping to dress the kids in their dive gear. The SEALs had watched the British divers carefully. Now, they could prepare the kids almost as well as the Brits did. They didn't miss a trick.

Every day, I was more impressed by these SEALs. They didn't say much, but they were amazingly dedicated and courageous gentlemen – and not just because they had signed on for this duty without the slightest idea how long it might last or how it might end. They didn't seek personal glory. As 'operators', they couldn't even share their names. But they looked after the Wild Boars (and the rest of us) with extraordinary care and compassion, twenty-four hours a day. They were cheerful. They were uncomplaining. They were competent and hugely fit. No task, no matter how challeng- ing or menial, was above or beneath them. More food. Another space blanket. An extra bottle of water for the night. If the SEALs had it, they would give it to the lads. They played games with the boys, creating a checkers board with rocks and dirt. None of the kids could beat the quick-thinking SEALs. And they did all this in an environment that was entirely foreign to them. Tham Luang was indeed in northern Thailand. But it might as well have been on the far side of the moon. The SEALs were strong divers. As the special- operations force of the Royal Thai Navy, they'd received the finest training their military could provide with hands-on assistance from their special-ops allies, the US Navy SEALs. But a flooded cave was not their natural habitat. From their base in the south-eastern province of Chonburi, they had trained in the open waters of the Bay of Bangkok at the northern end of the Gulf of Thailand. Cave diving was new to them.

The three SEALs in chamber 9 with Pak and the boys were part of a much-larger SEAL presence at the scene. More than 125 current and former Thai SEALs had joined the mission, many of them manning the forward-operating base that chamber 3 had become.

And let's not forget: the Thai Navy SEALs were the one and only organisation that had actually suffered a fatality during the Thai-cave rescue with the death of their former first-class petty officer Saman Gunan.

We'd made a decision not to tell the boys about Saman's death, the same way we had decided to shield the boys from any bad news about their teammates. Why upset the kids? But many of the SEALs did know Saman personally, his family too. I doubt many of these men were fully aware of the grave dangers they faced in the cave. That may well have been true of Petty Officer Gunan. Though he hadn't done much diving in the twelve years since he'd retired and had little if any experience in caves, he and his brothers all had the hearts of heroes. He retained all his fitness and his gung-ho spirit – and responded immediately to the call for volunteers. He was an undeniably brave and selfless man.

It might have been nice, actually, if the SEALs had spent a little more time thinking about their own safety and wellbeing. It was Jason who first brought up the issue of the SEALs and their gas. 'You guys have enough gas to get yourselves out of here after we're done?' he asked.

No experienced cave diver would ever swim into a cave without being certain he had sufficient air in his tanks to swim back out. That's Cave Diving Rule Number 1. But Jason's question was met with a moment of silence as Pak and the SEALs consulted among themselves.

'Actually, no, we don't,' Pak said. And they were short at least one face mask.

Though they'd rushed into the cave to be helpful, it seemed they had never really considered the details of getting out.

'When were you going to tell us this?' Rick asked under his breath. If we hadn't checked, would they have brought it up at all?

Rick told Pak not to worry. When the divers returned the next morning, we would bring in fresh air tanks for the SEALs and plant some extras on the route out, just in case. 'We're not leaving you in here,' Rick promised.

And what about Coach Ekk? I was still hoping to anaesthetise as few of these guys as possible.

I put it to Pak. 'Instead of sedating the coach and diving him out with the boys, why don't you and the SEALs swim out with him the normal way at the end?' I asked. 'He's a grown-up. I'm not sure we really need to sedate him.'

The more I'd thought about it, the more I liked the idea of letting Ekk come out with Pak and the SEALs. It would cut our third-day rescue count from five to four. Four was already a lot for the British divers. They weren't complaining, but I wasn't keen on adding an extra trip. Plus, if I could get out of sedating another patient, that was fine with me. I'd still be sedating a dozen of them. At some point, I knew, I'd be pressing my luck. Ekk was a 25-year-old. With a little instruction, couldn't he handle the dive? He'd have Pak and the SEALs at his side the whole way. If anything went wrong, they'd be right there.

'He'll be fine,' I assured Pak. 'See what he thinks.'

The Thai military doctor agreed to discuss my suggestion with the coach. Pak made no predictions, but he said he'd get back to me on it. When he did, the answer was unequivocal.

'Absolutely not,' Pak quoted Coach Ekk as telling him. 'He's been watching you take these kids out asleep. He likes the way it's going. He said thank you, but he wants to go out exactly the same way.'

So much for that idea.

*

Jason made the first trip out that day. He had Mick, real name Panumas Saengdee. At thirteen, he was one of the younger boys on the soccer team, though you wouldn't know it by watching him play. Mick was bigger than the other kids his age and a speed demon across the pitch. His coaches marvelled that he had the ball-handling skills of an athletic fifteen-year-old. Because of Mick's strength in the air and his agile head skills, the coaches considered playing him as a striker, though he ended up as a defender. As soon as he got out of the cave and home to his family, he might have some explaining to do. A student at Mae Sai Prasitsart, Mick never told his mum and dad he was going to Tham Luang. He thought they'd never give him permission.

I loved learning the back stories of these boys. In so much of the media coverage, they were just 'the players,' 'the boys' or 'the Wild Boars'. Like any group of young people, they had strong and distinct personalities – and bundles of charm. I was slowly getting to know them. It was hard to look at them and not think of my own wonderful children, who are also as distinct and colourful as can be. I think they trained me for these kids. But again there were questions when Jason and Mick reached the field hospital. 'Which one is he? Which one is he?' Just as I had with the boys on the first day, I failed to label him. I had brought the wristbands with me, but they disappeared during the swim in. I wouldn't get this right until the third day.

John Volanthen was up next. He took fourteen-year-old midfielder and left defender Adul Samon, recognised by his fellow players as the team brainiac. He speaks five languages, plays three musical instruments and earns top marks as an eighth-grader at Ban Wiang Phan School. His language ability (Thai, Mandarin, Burmese, English and Wa) had been a huge plus when Rick and

John first came upon the boys in the cave. As the only reasonable English speaker, it was Adul who was able to communicate for the stranded boys. He was distinct in at least two other notable ways. He was the only Christian on a team of young Buddhists, and his family was stateless, a challenging status he shared with Coach Ekk. Adul's family came from a poor hill tribe in Myanmar's self-governing Wa region. He was taken in by the Mae Sai Grace Church when he was seven years old. Soccer wasn't his only sport. For two years in a row, his volleyball team had finished second in all of northern Thailand.

Next up was Biw, guided by Chris Jewell. Real name Ekkarat Wongsookchan, Biw is 'the Smiler'. The fourteen-year-old goal-keeper, a student at Darunratwitthaya School, had the sunniest disposition on the team. He was cheerful in victory. He was cheerful in defeat. He was even cheerful at the end of a gruelling practice, happily collecting all the soccer equipment. Once trapped in the cave, no one was surprised that Biw considered lifting the spirits of others to be his own personal mission.

I didn't want to get overconfident with these boys or our own ability to dive them out. The best way to avoid trouble, I figured, was just to stay focused on the here and now. Calm them down. Get them ready. Send them out. In my medical practice back home, I seldom performed the same procedure so many times in a row. It had its advantages.

We had dispatched seven already. We were onto number eight. Rick would ferry him out.

Somehow, I lost my glasses in the cave, which was stupid of me, I know. I needed them to read the tiny writing on the syringes. I certainly didn't want to give the drugs out of order or use a little-kid dose on a big kid and have him wake up before he even reached

Craig in chamber 8. And I couldn't borrow Rick's because, in my first glasses-related mishap of the day, I had sat on them and broken them that morning during our pre-dive meeting. What is it with me and glasses? I have no idea. All I know is that as Rick and I were getting the next boy ready to go, I looked in Rick's direction and noticed he was executing the same pinhole-vision manoeuvre as I was, rolling his index finger into a tight circle and peeking through the tiny opening in the middle.

'Look at us,' Rick laughed.

'Pathetic,' I agreed. 'A couple of blind, middle-aged men.'

But you know what? These middle-aged men were getting it done.

Rick's boy this time was Duangphet Promthep, nickname Dom. Thirteen years old when he went into the cave, he'd turned fourteen on 3 July. Dom wasn't only a powerful striker and the highest goal-scorer on the team, a pint-sized version of his idol, Manchester United striker Marcus Rashford. He was also team captain, an impressive recognition for someone his age. Another Mae Sai Prasitsart student, Dom was a natural motivator, respected by his teammates. He was without a doubt one of the more talented players on the team, even invited to the junior trials for two of the leading provincial teams, Sukhothai FC and Chiangrai United FC.

As I said my goodbyes to Pak and the SEALs for the night, I had no idea how today's four boys had fared once they'd left us. I knew they were well sedated when they departed chamber 9. I knew they were in the hands of world-class cave divers. But beyond that, like the night before, I knew nothing. Despite my growing confidence about the system we'd put in place, I didn't fool myself for a minute. They faced an endless array of potential perils along the way.

I assumed that if Craig had confronted any major problems in chamber 8, I'd have heard something by now. With the fuller staffing in the cave, we did have extra divers who could deliver a message back to me. Though I didn't hear anything, I still couldn't be sure if the silence was a sign of success or just silence.

'See you tomorrow, Dr Harry,' Pak said to me as I prepared to slide into the water to swim out for the night, leaving him behind in the cave with three SEALs, four boys and a 25-year-old assistant coach.

I'd told him I'd be back, but would I really?

The way he said it – 'see you tomorrow' – caught me off guard. It was just an expression, something people say without a second thought. But there was a tone in Pak's voice. Was it hopefulness? Wishful thinking? Was he saying the words out loud to make sure they came true? It had to be disconcerting, perhaps downright terrifying, to watch the divers all leave for the night as he and the others remained behind.

What would happen if the rains blew in? What other unknowns were out there? Would we really be back like we said?

'See you tomorrow, mate,' I answered.

Once out of the cave, we had a quick debrief with the British divers. Everyone agreed that the extra hands had made a big difference in the cave and that the second day had been a smoother operation than the first. The quicker pace was nice too, though I had to kick myself for screwing up the wristbands again. The early report on the second-day's boys – *whoever they might have been!* – was entirely positive. A couple of them were already on their way to the big hospital in Chiang Rai, we were told. After the debrief, Craig and

I plopped ourselves down in the Australian tent for a few minutes of relaxation with the AFP guys before we'd head back to the hotel to collapse. For dinner, we had pizza and Gatorade.

Then, amid some sudden stirring, someone said excitedly, 'The prime minister is coming.' Then, someone else said, 'The prime minister is coming. You have to stay around to meet him.'

Really?

Frankly, at that moment I couldn't even name the prime minister of the Kingdom of Thailand, even though I'd been in his country for several days by then and had a temporary licence to practise medicine there. But I nodded knowingly when one of the AFP guys leaned over to me and whispered, 'Prayut Chan-o-cha,' which I took to be the prime minister's name. 'He's a retired general.' Apparently, he'd been PM since 2014. 'He's taken quite an interest in the rescue,' I was told. 'He wants to come and shake your hand.'

It wasn't just me. It was the other divers too. 'You all have to line up, and he will shake your hands.'

So how was I getting out of this?

I found Michael Costa, our trusty DFAT handler. 'We've got to get out of here,' I told him. 'If I don't get some sleep, I'm not going to be able to function tomorrow.'

Craig was even more direct. 'This is just bullshit, having all these meetings,' he said. 'We need to get home and get to bed. In the future, Harry can just brief somebody else, and they can give our report at whatever meetings they have going on. They can meet the prime minister. This isn't safe for anybody, keeping us up all night then going into the cave for another ten hours the next day.'

Michael sounded sympathetic, but his sympathy ran headlong into a late-breaking fact. 'Oh, my God,' he said, 'the road's been closed by security because the prime minister is coming up.'

I couldn't believe we were really stuck.

'So how do we get out?' I asked Michael.

That's when I had the single greatest plan that I've ever created, a true moment of genius.

'All right,' I said to Michael. 'I know what we do. We all get into one of those ambulances. We put the flashing lights on, and we go down the hill. Can you organise it?'

Michael hesitated, but for only a second. Then he too was over-whelmed by the obvious brilliance of my plan.

'Okay,' he said. 'Let's try.'

Michael went off and found one of the Thai medical people and said: 'We need an ambulance at once. The Australian doctors must get home to bed, and the only way out of here is in an ambulance.'

The answer came back straightaway: *Whatever Dr Harry needs.*

Michael led us – more like *snuck* us – through the dark to where the ambulances were parked. From there, we had a clear view of the road out, which was all lit up for the prime minister's arrival with soldiers lined up on either side.

'Craig,' I said, 'you jump in the back and I'll jump in the front.' I think he got the better spot.

He opened the sliding door on the side of the ambulance, and who was sitting there in the light? Ten Thai nurses, each of them more beautiful than the others. I took out my phone and began taking pictures of Craig and the nurses. Soon, the Thai nurses were giggling, hugging Craig, posing for photos and bringing out their own phones.

'*Woo hoo!*' Craig called out as the ambulance pulled onto the main road. We flew past the security barriers and the lines of soldiers, through the cover of darkness back to our border-side hotel.

Much as I would have liked to shake the hand of the Thai prime minister, it was a flash of true genius, I have to say at the risk of repeating myself.

I think even Craig was proud of me. I know Heather appreciated it when I texted some of the nurse photos back to her in Perth.

22

Old Boy

Harry

I got down to breakfast on Tuesday morning before Craig did. When he arrived a couple of minutes later, he stopped at the buffet, filled a large bowl with noodles, then came over and joined me. Both of us were eager to fuel up well for the big day ahead. If the cheerful news was that we kept getting better at this, we also faced fresh challenges. On this, the third day of the rescue, we'd be trying to dive out with four boys *and* the coach, five altogether. And everyone was expecting us to succeed.

'Imagine if we kill someone today,' Craig said.

'It will be even worse than losing one on the first day, now that the expectations are so high,' I agreed. 'Everyone will be asking, "How did you screw up so badly?" Any failure will be totally our fault.'

'How quickly things change,' Craig allowed. 'All of a sudden, no one wants to believe this is hard.'

It's like childbirth in the modern era. A hundred years ago, when women regularly died having babies, those deaths were almost expected. Today, dying in childbirth is so uncommon, people immediately want to know: 'What did the doctor do wrong?'

It wasn't hard to understand why the confidence was up in the stratosphere. Eight boys were safely in Chiangrai Prachanukroh Hospital, all of them, as far as we knew, doing fine. They might even be eating ice cream. The breathless news updates were flying every minute or two. The 'Miracle in the Cave' headlines – as if any of this were a miracle and not a result of plain old human effort and ingenuity – were blasting around the world. In just a few hours, everyone sounded certain, all the boys would be out of the cave.

The politicians seemed to agree. Why else would the Thai prime minister come to congratulate the rescuers on a mission – the ones willing to hang around and meet him – that wasn't even complete yet? Why else would Governor Narongsak Osottanakorn, the rescue coordinator, tell a packed press conference: 'For the next rescue we believe we can do even better and that it will be a 100 per cent success.'

'Now all we have to do is convince ourselves,' Craig said.

Just then, a man and a woman came over and joined us at the table. They were part of the Australian Federal Police team, who were also staying in the hotel. But these two weren't police officers, as they quickly made clear. He was a chaplain named Steve Neuhaus. She was Roz Brown, a psychologist. Apparently, they travel often on AFP missions to look after everyone's spiritual and mental wellbeing. Since we were part of this mission, their concern naturally extended to us.

Neither Craig nor I are at all religious, and neither of us felt any need for counselling at that moment. I hope we'd both be open to asking for that kind of help if we felt we needed it, though we would definitely want to be the ones to ask. Craig, if anything, was even more resistant than I was.

So, of course, the chaplain turned to Craig.

'Craig,' he said, leaning forwards in his seat, 'how are you feeling this morning?'

Craig didn't let half a second of silence hover in the air.

'This morning, Father,' he responded firmly, 'I'm feeling like a man of science.'

And that was it. Father Steve went back to his cup of tea, obviously deflated. Our counselling session was done.

The walk into the cave that morning was more sombre than usual. As Craig, Rick, John and I proceeded quietly together, I could tell the Brits were feeling unhappy. It had rained overnight. There was talk of more rain to come. And there was something else too: a general sense that time was moving past us, that conditions in the cave were worsening, that despite our best efforts we really might have missed the boat. Rick and John had been there early enough to see the cave in full flood, swirling brown rapids that drove even the fittest and most skilled divers back, threatening to pin them into a crevice or under a ledge. No one wanted to die that way and certainly not after two days of success. I respected the experience of these guys highly enough to know that if they were worried, I should be worried too. John seemed especially out of sorts, verbalising his fears that the water levels in the cave were starting to rise. It was undermining my confidence. At an opportune rest break in the dry-cave section, we stopped to quickly talk it through.

'What's up, you blokes?' I asked. 'Is this safe or not? You guys have the experience in this cave. What do you want to do?'

It was Rick who spoke up. 'Let's look at the water-level device in the next chamber,' he said. 'If it's risen, that could mark the start of significant flooding. If it's okay, we proceed. If there is any sense that water is rising at any stage inside the cave, we bail out and come straight out. Even one centimetre change. Agreed?'

Craig wasn't so sure. He took the view that if the water levels did rise, we would still be able to get out with the flow, even if we couldn't get through to chamber 9. He thought John was going a bit over the top. But we ultimately agreed to err on the side of Rick's cautious recommendation. We caught up with Chris and Jason. They agreed.

Luckily the water rose no more.

That morning, several of the divers, including Craig and I, had decided to take extra cylinders with us. That way, the SEALs would have plenty of gas for even a slow dive out. It was hard to say how long the trip might take them. Given their newness to cave diving, we didn't expect any speed records. On the way in, they'd taken twice as long to reach the boys as Rick and John had, breathing their way through most of the four cylinders they swam in with. However quickly they got out, they'd need to breathe along the way, and now they would be able to.

'I would recommend you dive out one at a time, not all bunched together,' I said to Pak once we made it back to chamber 9. He shared this advice with the others. 'Leave plenty of space between each man. As you know, there are some tight spots out there. You don't want to crash into each other. It will be far smoother if you go one at a time. Also, wait a couple of hours after I leave, so the water clears up for you.' If there was a problem with any of the boys on the way out that caused a hold-up, I didn't want extra divers piling up behind them to complicate the situation. Frankly, I also didn't want the SEALs anywhere near me when I was making my own exit at the end of the day.

One diver at a time had worked well so far in the rescue. There was no reason it wouldn't also work well for the SEALs.

They listened carefully to my explanation with their usual polite respect. They spoke earnestly among themselves. Then, Pak delivered the verdict. 'I don't think so,' he said. 'We are a team. We will come out together as a team. That is what they say.'

Since we had five Wild Boars to rescue today, we had to make some adjustments in the diver line-up. Jason would take the first one, whomever that turned out to be – but only as far as chamber 8. There, he would meet up with Jim Warny, who would ferry that one out the rest of the way. Jason would then swim back to chamber 9 and handle the fifth (and final) trip of the day. John, Rick and Chris would ferry the second, third and fourth.

Got all that? Yes, it was a little complicated and, as the day got rolling, it would get even more so. There were a few other issues that also needed to be resolved. One was labelling the boys with their names. I was going to make it happen this time, I swore to myself. I wouldn't mess with wristbands any more. I brought a waterproof marker along, and I would get the SEALs to write each boy's name on his arm. I'd been a slow learner on this. But the third time, I told myself, really would be a charm.

There was also an issue with the face masks. We had only four of the style that we had been using for the previous two days, masks that we knew were a good size and effective for the boys. We would take the next best two other masks with us to give us some options. We'd have to figure that out on the fly. But we were all finally in position, and now we were ready to go.

I didn't know ahead of time which of the boys I'd be sending out of the cave first today, but I had assumed one thing: Coach Ekk would be the last one out, even though he had declined my gentle suggestion that he swim out under his own power with the SEALs. Like the captain on a sinking ship, Coach Ekk would naturally usher his players out before him. By now, the whole world knew how much he cared about them. No one ever told me he'd come out last. I just expected it. In a final gesture of gracious leadership, the young, inspiring assistant soccer coach, anaesthetised or not, would insist on hitting the water last.

That's how it always goes in the movies, right? Women and children first! Well, it was the third day of the rescue at Tham Luang cave, and life wouldn't quite imitate art this time.

When the day's first young traveller came down the slope, he was suited up like all the rest of them in a small-size wetsuit, buoyancy collar and hood. He had the bungees around his mid-section and the cable ties on his wrists. John helped me prepare him for the trip.

'Hello, little fella,' I said brightly as the youngster settled onto my knee and I continued with the preparations for his long journey ahead. 'How are you feeling today?'

'Okay,' he said softly.

'I'm gonna jab you a couple of times – good boy, good boy.'

He wasn't too chatty, but I was going strong, and Pak was there to translate when I needed him. I patted my young patient on the shoulder. With my usual banter, I tried to distract him from the two needles he was about to receive. I cuddled him and tried to be soothing. It wouldn't be much longer, I knew, until he slipped into sweet unconsciousness.

'How old are you?' I asked.

'Twenty-five,' he answered.

I thought he was messing with me.

'Oh, yeah,' I said with a smile. 'I'm twenty-five too. Just turned twenty-five.

'And what position do you play on the soccer team?' Pak was translating for both of us.

'Coach,' the answer came back.

'I am a famous soccer coach back in Australia,' I said, playing along with the obvious ruse.

'No, really, Dr Harry,' Pak interrupted. 'He's the coach. Coach Ekk.'

'*Bullshit!*' I sputtered, flustered but laughing at my screw-up. John, who was holding the face mask, smiled and shook his head at me. 'You idiot, Harry.' In the background, the ever-efficient Jason was getting geared up for the trip.

It was only then that I looked closely under the boy's diving hood, which apparently I had neglected to do before. He wasn't a boy at all. Damned if I didn't now see a few wispy hairs growing out of his 25-year-old chin.

Oops!

In my defence, the coach was definitely smaller than a couple of his players. I didn't have a chance to weigh anyone, but I'd put him around sixty kilos. Two, maybe three of the boys, were more like sixty-five.

I'm not sure if the coach thought any of that was funny. I'm not even sure if he grasped my mistake. As for his decision to come out first on this final day of the rescue, maybe he was afraid we would forget him. Maybe he was just a tad suspicious given the earlier talk about him swimming out conscious with the SEALs. But Pak, John and I all got a smile out of my embarrassing misidentification.

'Ready for a jab, mate?' I asked in my best, deep, blokey voice to the grown man who was still sitting on my lap.

After Jason headed into the water with the youthful coach and made the planned hand-off to Jim Warny, Jason would start his swim back to chamber 9 so he'd be in position for his second dive of the day. But John was up next. I waited a decent interval – no more traffic jams, please – before asking Pak to send the next one down the hill. He turned out to be the big boy, sixteen-year-old defender Phonchai Khamluang, nickname Tee. A studious pupil at the Ban Pa Yang School, Tee was the largest of the Wild Boars. Quiet, tidy, eager to work hard, he is a member of the school council and a volunteer traffic director outside the building as students arrive each morning. Like Coach Ekk and two of the other boys, he is stateless. Tee and his family are Tai Yai, members of a marginalised tribe originally from Shan state in neighbouring Myanmar. That has made life difficult for the family any time they have tried to find work, own property and travel away from home.

Jab, jab, dress and go: By now, this little system of ours was running like a well-oiled machine. If practice made perfect, we were getting better every time. This was the third trip for each of the British divers. Pak, the SEALs and I had even more experience. It was easy to forget how recently our success had seemed so unlikely and our approach so reckless. No more. I had finally begun to believe we just might achieve the impossible.

'Next,' I called out to Pak, signalling I was ready to keep it going.

Over the past two days, the chatter up on the ledge had grown noticeably quieter. We'd started with thirteen Wild Boars, and now only three boys remained. Suddenly, I heard a burst of laughter mixed with a collision of raised voices. In the darkness, I called up to Pak, hoping he would clue me in.

The Thai doctor always seemed to have a smile on his face. But when he came to the side of the ledge and looked down at me, he almost seemed to be giggling. The SEALs, he explained, had caught the boys stuffing American MREs into their wetsuits, preparing to smuggle the military rations out of the cave with them.

'They like the flavours,' he said. 'Very much. They have a new favourite food.'

Rick would dive out with the boy known as Titan, Chanin Wiboonrungrueang, at eleven the youngest Wild Boar. A forward on the soccer team, Titan was in his final year at Anubanmaesai primary school and lives near Thailand's border with Myanmar. When he was ten, he spent time as a schoolboy monk, and photos of his shaven head and saffron robes still hung in the family home. Though his grandmother, Yod Kantawong, is stateless and his hairdresser mother was born in Myanmar, his mum married a salesman from Thailand and after three years became eligible for Thai citizenship. So Titan was born a Thai citizen, free to ride his bicycle back and forth across the border and visit relatives on both sides. Sadly, his grandmother enjoyed no such privilege. When her grandson went missing, she had to apply for a special visitor's slip to rush across the border. Titan and his family were very close to Coach Ekk. When his parents were away, Titan often stayed with Ekk and his aunt.

The first three dives of the day – Coach Ekk's, Tee's and Titan's – all went like clockwork. Practice really was making perfect, as it usually does. We should probably teach a course in this, I thought to myself. But we still had two boys to go in this great cave rescue of ours. Nothing is ever finished till it's finished. As it turned out, we weren't even close to done.

Chris Jewell would dive out with thirteen-year-old Somphong Jaiwong, Pong to his friends. A right-winger and midfielder on the team and a student at Mae Sai Prasitsart, Pong was one of those boys who always made sure his friends were comfortable, happy and having a good time. He had an alarm on his watch that he set for 6 a.m. and noon, letting all the others know if it was day or night outside.

Pong was raised by his Uncle Chai after his father died. 'He's football mad and spends all his spare time playing or watching,' Uncle Chai marvelled. 'He was watching the World Cup with me before this.' Added his teacher, Manutsanun Kuntun: 'He dreams of becoming a footballer for the Thai national team.' And he had shown some talent too. Outside the cave, Uncle Chai posed proudly with the string of medals the boy had won playing soccer with his pals.

Such moving, human stories. Now, Pong was finally on his way home.

For three straight days, Mark, real name Mongkol Boonpiam, thought he was about to leave. He'd bravely volunteered to be one of the first to put on the diving gear and make the long journey out. He was fasted on day one in anticipation of his exit, before we knew how many boys a day we could handle. When Mark didn't make it out the first day, he was told he'd most likely depart on day two. When that didn't happen either, he was bumped to the third day – and now would finally be leaving, the last boy out of the cave on the very last day of the rescue.

Mark was another stateless boy, though he did have some hope of eventually earning Thai citizenship. Mark's parents were born in Myanmar. But they had lived in Thailand for ten years already, and he was born there. He had done what he could to leave a positive impression on his teachers and classmates. A bright, athletic seventh-grader at Ban Pa Muat School, he studied with almost the same enthusiasm he brought to swimming, cycling, volleyball and, especially, soccer. He'd been playing soccer since he was in kindergarten and loved the sport so much he was rarely seen without a football shirt. He was on the same volleyball team as his Wild Boar teammate Adul.

At thirteen years old, Mark was listed on the team roster as trainee. He wasn't the youngest boy on the team. But he was easily the tiniest, and that created one last complication for him. We didn't have a decent mask small enough. What we did have was a tiny pink child's mask, little more than a toy. But that seemed impossibly fragile to be safe. It also lacked the all-important positive-pressure function that we had come to rely on. The other option was a full-sized, grey, AGA commercial-diver's mask designed for a large adult man.

When the time came for the last child to leave, I called for him in the usual manner. I was shocked to see such a diminutive figure, all dressed in dive gear, come wobbling down the slope. Why was he so tiny? I thought we had sent out the smallest of the kids already. That's why we'd held back the two odd masks until last. And here I was now, faced with what appeared to be the smallest of them all!

'Who's this?' I asked Pak in horror. 'What's his weight?'

'Mark is his name,' Pak told me. 'He was thirty kilos when he came in.'

The boy standing in front of me looked far smaller than thirty kilograms. He was the smallest by far. And we had only the two untested masks to use. We had no choice. For all I knew, the rain was now bucketing down outside, and all our lives were in significant danger. Mark had to leave the cave, and he had to leave today.

I cracked on and injected his leg with ketamine, adjusting the dose for his delicate stature. Minutes later, he was asleep, and Jason stepped forwards, initially proffering the positive-pressure AGA. There was just no way. It was gaping all around Mark's little face. I could easily put my fingers in the gap between the mask seal and his cheek. That would never keep the water out or the air in. We tried the little pink mask. Time was ticking by, and we had to get the mask to seal. With no positive pressure, any trickle of water into the mask could easily drown the boy. The soft, silicone skirt seemed horribly delicate. The whole mask was just flopping around. After ten minutes of refitting, padding out Mark's face with foam and getting the best seal possible, Jason looked into my eyes. We realised we could do no more. If we mucked around further, Mark would get dangerously hypothermic and would need another top up of ketamine. It was now or never. So close to total success, we were looking at certain disaster.

It was up to Jason now. All he could do was dive Mark out. Once he started, he would have to keep moving, finally appearing at chamber 3 with a tiny corpse or a living boy. My heart sank for the hundredth time as the pair swam down the canal towards home.

23

Last Out

Harry

I began what I knew would be my final dive out. Moving with the current, kicking as I went, hand over hand, methodically down the line. My fourth day in the water, I was finally feeling like I had built some mastery over Tham Luang. Craig was up ahead of me. Mikko and Claus were with him. Chris and Jason were up there somewhere with their boys. Jim and the Coach, Rick's kid and John's kid, I told myself, should already be at the field hospital by now. Everyone was heading in the same direction.

Out. All the way out.

Only Pak and the SEALs remained behind in chamber 9.

I stopped briefly to say hello to a couple of the guys still waiting at their assigned stations. Erik was just sitting in the mud with his thoughts. I stopped and had a chat with him.

'Which part of Canada are you from, mate?' I asked. 'Craig and I will be over there in September caving in Alberta. I imagine it will be a bit different to this, eh?'

He seemed like a great guy. Calm. Solid. Unshaken by the previous days' events.

On I swam, wanting to distance myself from the combat swimmers who'd be following.

As I moved through the relative ease of chamber 4, I steeled myself for what I knew was still waiting for me, the final, tough section of the cave, the tightly constricted passage connecting chambers 4 and 3. But even before I got there, I heard a voice in the darkness ahead of me.

'Harry? Harry? Is that you?'

It was Chris. I recognised him immediately. He sounded distressed. Not a tone I expected to hear in his voice.

'Yeah,' I called back. 'Are you all right? Is the kid okay?'

'The kid's fine,' Chris answered. 'It's me. Come down if you can.'

As quickly as I was able to kick and pull, I raced down the line towards Chris. There he was in the water with the kid floating next to him, face down, bubbling happily away. But Chris looked white as a sheet.

'I dropped the line,' he said. 'I've been lost for fifteen minutes. I got all turned around.'

I had never seen Chris in this state before. The man is super cool and highly experienced. But as he explained it to me, he'd just had the nearest near-miss a cave diver can have. And it happened at the nastiest, narrowest part of the cave.

Before he and Pong got this far, Chris said, Jason and his boy, Mark, had caught up to them. Jason, I believe, helped Chris top up Pong, who appeared to be rousing and needed another dose. Jason and Mark then moved ahead of them, flipping the order of the last two teams out. Chris and Pong had been the second last to leave me in chamber 9. Now, they'd be the final pair exiting the cave.

In this section, the line is on your left side. At one point there is a classic line trap, where the line goes into a section that is too small for a human to follow. You have to extend your arm out to hold the line as it gets pulled around a left-hand corner. At that point, the cave is really narrow before it opens up again, and you need to fit your body through a small vertical slot. Feeling far to the right, you find the slot and try get through it without letting go of the line on your left. It is almost an unsolvable puzzle on your own. Add an anaesthetised child to the equation, and it is amazing there hadn't already been an accident here. You're doing it all with your eyes closed – or you might as well be. With so much traffic through the cave now, the silt was everywhere. There was no underwater visibility. Zero. You're pulling the line as you swim through the cave. The problem is, it's very easy to drop it. If you did, suddenly, you would find yourself wondering, *Oh, shit. Where's the line gone?*

Apparently, that's exactly what happened to Chris.

He had been searching desperately for the line and couldn't find it. All he'd found so far was an electrical cable on the floor of the cave. *This has to go somewhere,* he reasoned. *I'll just follow it out.* Unfortunately, he followed the cable in the opposite direction, deeper into the cave. When he finally surfaced, he wasn't sure where he was: In chamber 4? In some side alcove? He couldn't even tell any more which way was in and which was out. He didn't have the guide line. He couldn't find it. He was truly lost.

Fifteen minutes in the dark with a limited supply of air and a sedated child who needs to get out of the cave – those minutes can feel like a lifetime, and not a very pleasant one. Chris was stranded in chamber 4, trying to gather himself, when he saw my light coming through.

'Okay,' I told him, 'no worries. You sit here. Take all the time you need. I will hand you the line. Let yourself calm down. Come out when you're ready. I'll take the kid through.'

Without a second of hesitation, Chris agreed. He passed the boy to me, and I took over from there.

I was secretly pleased to be able to escort one of the anaesthetised kids through part of the cave. Across three draining days, I had been sedating them, prepping them for their risky journeys and passing them off to Rick, John, Jason and Chris. Now, after all that, I would finally get to dive one of the kids out myself. I didn't wish Chris any difficulty. He's a fine man, and I have huge respect for him as a cave diver. That said, I did also feel like I was missing out on part of the Thai cave-rescue experience. I didn't want to make this about me or us, and it wasn't. It was about the boys. But I'd be lying if I didn't acknowledge that on some level I was also happy to have my crack at the part I hadn't experienced yet. I'd been looking after the kids all this time. Now, I thought to myself, it will feel like I've done a bit of everything.

How little I knew about how far *everything* went.

I pulled the kid close to me and got a firm hold of the line. Together, we started moving along the same path that Chris had. We got to the exact spot where Chris came unstuck, the super-tight passage where chamber 4 leads into chamber 3. It's a dicey part of the cave, I knew that – maybe the most dicey. So I approached with extra care.

I'd better have a reach over here with my left hand, I said to myself, *and keep my other hand on the kid while I hold onto the line at the same time.* But I only had two hands. So I grabbed the line and placed it under the crook of my arm, holding it securely in my armpit. What could be safer than that? Then, I proceeded to do the other things I needed to do to slip the both of us through the narrow opening.

My main task was to change sides with the boy, readjusting our positions so we could both get through this hole.

I knew exactly what this entailed. The precise manoeuvre was etched in my mind. We were right beside each other, the boy and me. His breathing was fine. We were lined up like we were supposed to be. I was ready to dive us through this narrow hole. Then, I thought: *Okay, where's the line?*

Where is it? I just had it. You are bloody joking. I can't find the line!

I took a breath. I steadied my composure. I still couldn't find the line. *You idiot! Exactly the same thing that just happened to Chris – and now it's happened to me!*

I did what twenty-five years of cave diving had taught me, starting with not losing my cool. *Stop, breathe, think, ACT.* I went into my lost-line search drill. I stayed right where I was. I tried not to move in any direction. I made sure I had a solid grip on the boy. I didn't want him floating off as I hunted for this missing line.

I made large circles with my arms. I felt nothing.

I swept across the hard roof of the cave. Nothing there.

I covered the limestone wall in front of me. Nothing there. I felt down on the floor. Still nothing.

If the line was out there, I was going to find it. I knew I would.

I forced myself to stay calm. Panic kills more divers than empty cylinders and falling rocks combined. The line had to be nearby.

I did the same thing on my left side. No line.

I did the same thing on my right. Still no line.

Fuck!

I could not find the line. I was sitting in the dark. We had to get out of there. Even with a top-up dose of ketamine, the kid wouldn't stay out forever. Chris was somewhere behind us. The time was chiming in my head like Big Ben.

I reached around on the floor again. This time, I felt something. It was electrical cable, possibly the same bit that Chris had found. My mind went to the same place that his did. *Oh, well, at least I know which way is out. I can follow the cable out rather than going back in.* That might work. Maybe it wouldn't. I was feeling stupid and frightened too.

Suddenly, I moved my arm, and there was the line.

It was in my armpit, exactly where it had been all this time.

I felt even more dopey, only now my feelings of stupidity were seasoned with deep relief. On the rest of the way out, I never let go of the rope again.

I did smack my head a few more times on the limestone. It was hard to avoid. The stalactites hung low and unpredictably in that part of the cave. I was trying to protect the boy. As we moved through the very narrowest stretch, I nestled him right under my chin. That kept him protected effectively but turned my head into a bit of a battering ram. I had my helmet on, but I still received a jarring blow every time I encountered another rock.

I went with the flow as well as I was able to. Once we got through the tightest part, we were scooting along the line very nicely, building up a bit of momentum as we closed in on chamber 3. I wanted to keep moving. I didn't want anything stopping us now. We had the water flow behind us. I was kicking with my fins, just following the line.

Bang! Bang! I whacked my helmet a couple of more times.

I kept my hand out in front of me, feeling as we went. There was no seeing anything. By this point, my neck was getting sore. I could swear it was also being shortened with every sharp bang. That couldn't have actually been happening – could it? – but I just kept thinking: *I may lose some brain cells before I get out of here, but I won't get lost and the kid will be delivered safely home.*

When I held my breath, I could hear him breathing. In and out. In and out. I could feel the bubbles coming up past my face. It was a soothing feeling. It was a fabulous sound. To me, the boy's steady breathing was a soaring vindication of all we had struggled to achieve. My arm around his belly could feel the movement with every breath. Everything felt right. But I'd had enough of this place.

It was the whirring of the electric pumps that told me how close we were to chamber 3.

There was hope in that sound but also a few tinges of nervousness. As the whirring got louder and my hand was still extended in front of me, the thought did occur: *I really don't want to put my fingers into those pump blades.* I assumed the pumps had screens on the front that were supposed to shield the suction part, protecting careless divers from allowing any of their extremities to get sliced off. But those pumps are massive and their suction power is fierce, and we were sharing the same cave water with them.

The sound was getting louder and louder as we swam closer in. If I dared, I am sure I could have reached out and touched one of those machines.

It seemed to take forever to go the last few metres. When I wasn't fixated on my fingers, I was still obsessed with the safety of the child.

Then suddenly, just like that, my head popped out of the water. I didn't realise I was there yet, but then I was. As my knees dug into the mud beneath me, the light in the chamber hit my eyes. It was bright. It made me squint. That's when I knew Pong and I were just about home.

In that flash, people were all over us. Yelling. Cheering. Laughing. Clapping their hands. Shouting 'All right!' and 'Way to go!' and 'You made it!' and all kinds of other stuff I couldn't comprehend.

The first hands I felt were those of three American pararescuers. They jumped into the water with us, these big, strong, fit guys.

'Hey, doc,' I heard one of them say. 'Well done, man!'

They were all patting me on the back. One of them grabbed the kid. In an instant, the boy was gone. Onto a stretcher. Through chamber 3. Out of the cave. Up the hill into the field hospital, where a team of Thai doctors and nurses was waiting for him. As he was heading away from me, he hadn't stirred at all.

'Is everyone all right?' I asked.

'You bet,' one of the Americans answered. 'They're all out. They're all fine.'

For a moment, things turned quiet in my head. I was trying to wrap my mind around everything that was happening. I understood that the results were all positive. I could tell that the people were happy and energised. But in that brief moment of silence, it was almost like I wasn't there. Or I was there, but I was staring down at me in the water and trying to make sense of it all.

That passed quickly. *Wow*, I thought to myself. *It's over. The job is done.* Unless something went wrong with one of the kids in the next half hour, everyone was going to be well. All I could do was climb out of the water and share the glorious feeling with those who had helped to make it so.

The crowd around me grew, and the faces clarified. Rick and the other British divers stepped forwards. Then there was Craig, flashing the biggest smile I had ever got from him. Without Craig, I knew, we never could have achieved all this and rescued these boys. We were a team, then and now. Chris was still behind me. I was sure he'd arrive shortly. Erik and some of the others began to appear. And soon, it seemed like almost everyone was there. The other American para-rescuers. The Chinese. The Thai military people and volunteers, the ones who had been manning chamber 3. They were standing around with giant smiles on their faces and climbing out of their wetsuits.

I have never won the lottery before, but I'll bet it doesn't feel any more exhilarating than this. I was nervous. I was numb. Then it hit me. And I realised a moment later my life will never again be the same.

I think it was Claus – it could have been Erik or one of the Americans – who pulled out a bottle of Jack Daniels. Someone found some paper cups. It was a special moment, and these were many of the people who had delivered it home, divers and other rescuers in the cave.

It was time for a toast.

To us.

We knew the whole world was watching. We knew what the odds were when we began. We knew how quickly we'd have been held responsible if anything had gone wrong. Now we had seen what our plan and our teamwork could achieve.

The bottle went around the circle. Everyone took a pour.

'To us,' the great Rick Stanton said as the little paper cups were raised in the air. 'And to the boys.' I swear even Jason Mallinson cracked a smile.

We lingered a while longer, soaking up each other's company. Someone passed around a bucket of KFC. No one seemed eager to leave.

Then Claus spoke up.

'You know,' he said, 'the SEALs are still in there, Dr Pak and his guys.'

That was true. They had spent more time in the cave by far than any of the rest of us had. They had signed on, promising to stay for as long as the boys did, when no one had any idea how long that might be. They had been so concerned about caring for the team that they had neglected to secure the gas they would need for their own dive out.

Exiting the cave was still a big dive for them. We didn't have to be reminded of that. Despite their special-ops training and their strong esprit de corps, the Thai SEALs' dive training was for open ocean. The cave environment was still head-shakingly unfamiliar territory for them.

We wouldn't consider us out of the cave until Pak and the SEALs were fully out too. That would take several more hours. Before they left chamber 9, Pak and the SEALs wanted to let the silt settle, and they wanted to avoid any human traffic jams. At least now they had the air to make the journey. It would have been easier if they had exited one by one or in pairs. But they were a team. They wanted to travel together. And they did. Finally, a few minutes before 11 p.m., everyone was out of the cave.

V

Living

24

Call Home

Harry

I texted Fiona as soon as Craig and I left the cave.

'All out,' I wrote, followed by: 'Might be having a few beers. Call you when back at the hotel.'

That had been our ritual on each of the past three nights, after our initial recon trip and after each of the first two rescue days. I would text Fiona as soon as I was safely outside, letting her know that all was well and I was back on solid ground. Craig checked in with Heather as well. He and I were always thoroughly exhausted. Both of us were desperately ready to sleep. But there were always things to be done before we could square away our gear, leave the cave site and ride the van back to the hotel for the night. It was a long list: debrief on the day's activities. Meet with the other divers to clear up any glitches. Talk through the latest suggestions from the Thai authorities. Check the medications for the next day. And we had to map out a plan for the following morning, learning from the previous day's experiences and trying to get better every time. What all that meant in practical terms was that on the previous three nights, it had taken a couple of hours to get back to the hotel and for me to get Fiona on the phone. Since Adelaide time was two and a half hours ahead of the time in Mae Sai, it was always late by the time we got to speak.

Fiona didn't seem to mind the hour. She wanted to hear my voice, to get the update and to know that I was alive, even if it meant cuddling up in her PJs for a couple of hours on the couch. And I was certainly eager to hear her voice. In just the past three nights, I had come to treasure those bleary phone chats. When your emotions are running as wild as mine were, having a calm, loving spouse to connect with, even on another continent, is about the closest thing to sanity you are likely to find. But on this night, the last night of rescue, the first night of celebration, I suspected our bedtime conversation might be even later than it had been before.

We had downed those paper cups of whiskey in chamber 3. We had walked the attaboy gauntlet of 'Congratulations! Thank you! It's a miracle!' The boys were finally safe and out of the cave. In the days to come, I knew, all of Thailand – the whole *world* – would find grand ways to celebrate. But in between all that, Craig and I just wanted to have a few quiet beers with our mates. With the pressure and the craziness we'd all been living with the past few days, this might be our only semi-normal opportunity to hang out and bond.

We stopped at the Australian tent. The AFP and DFAT guys had been all about following the rules in Thailand. Now, even they were ready to move past the dry-mission policy and blow the froth off a couple of coldies. From some darkened corner of the tent, one of them retrieved a carton of beer, which we did our best to deal with. Someone else ordered a pizza. Who knew there were pizza deliveries to Tham Luang cave? I guess we shouldn't have been surprised. A whole city had grown up here over the past two weeks. The pizza-delivery woman was so excited that the boys were out, she lingered for a couple of beers herself.

The rain had set in consistently now. And here's the great part of that: it didn't matter. Everyone was out of the cave. Just a few hours earlier, rain could have been a catastrophe. Now, who cared?

Nothing especially brilliant or insightful was said, not that I can recall. It was more like, 'Can you believe this is over?' and 'We really did it' and 'Wow!' It was really just a well-earned, two-hour Aussie exhale, our own private moment, a chance for some homegrown heroes to take it all in.

Even heading down the path to the van, we wouldn't escape the congratulations. It seemed like they'd go on forever. For the first time in my life, my hands were actually sore from having them vigorously shaken by so many enthusiastic well-wishers.

Meanwhile, more than 7000 kilometres away, a drama had been unfolding back in Adelaide that I knew nothing about. In fact, it had been unfolding for the past couple of days.

On Sunday night, after the first four boys were out of the cave, my eldest sister, Amanda, came by our house. She told Fiona that, the previous evening, my dad had had a bit of a wobbly episode at the nursing home. One of the nurses called an ambulance. Amanda went up to the hospital expecting the worst, thinking she might be seeing our father for the very last time. But he rallied, and the next day, he was up and dressed and back in his room at Regis Burnside, seeming totally fine.

'Manda,' Fiona said, 'you should have told me sooner. I could have done something.'

It had all happened so quickly, Amanda said. 'No one knew what was going on, and I didn't want to worry you.'

Crisis averted. Lucky too – because my sister Kristina and her husband, Jim, were also overseas at the time.

Then, on Tuesday night, as soon as Fiona had heard from me that the coach and the final boys were out of the cave and so were Craig and I, she texted Amanda, sharing the great news. 'Harry's out. Everyone's fine. We can all relax now.'

Amanda texted back immediately. 'I'm just going to pop round for a hug.' It was nearly eleven by then. When Amanda and her husband, Richard, arrived at the house a few minutes later, Fiona was emotionally spent, like everyone was. But she was already relieved beyond words. Didn't this moment call for a toast?

'It's finished,' Fiona said. 'They're all safe. I think I should open a bottle of champagne.'

'Let's just sit down,' Amanda said.

The three of them settled onto the couch in the family room. Amanda was the first to speak.

'Fi,' she said, hesitantly. 'I've got something else to tell you.'

Fiona knew straightaway what it was going to be. Or she thought she did. My dad was eighty-eight. He'd just had a health scare. But in the emotional swirl of the moment, another thought popped into Fiona's head. *Maybe it's Harry.* It wasn't.

'Dad died,' Amanda said.

The two women had a big hug. Amanda and Richard said how happy they were that the boys were out and I was okay. No one lingered long. They said their goodnights, leaving Fiona alone for one of the toughest conversations she'd ever have to have.

The thought had already occurred to Fiona: *Now, I've got to give Harry the news, whenever it is he calls.*

Our older son James had already gone to sleep. He had to work early in the morning. Our daughter, Millie, was in America. She had a summer job at Camp Jewell YMCA in Connecticut. Fiona would have liked to have had her daughter to talk to. Fiona went in and told our younger son Charlie that his papa had died and gave him a hug.

Fi knew it might be a while before she got the call from me, especially on this night. How long would 'might be having a few beers' take? That was hardly a precise measure of time. And what shape would I be in when she finally got me on the phone? How many beers *exactly*?

Maybe, she thought, it would be better to wait until morning to break the news. I could enjoy my night of celebration. Wouldn't all of this be a whole lot easier in the light of day?

But then, another thought occurred to her, and it was impossible to dismiss: *I don't want him finding out on Facebook or TV. I have to tell him tonight.*

It was 11.30 p.m. Thai time, two in the morning in Adelaide, when I finally got back to the hotel. I was sure Fiona would still be waiting up for me.

Craig had the room next to mine. Before he went to bed, he was eager to take a shower, but his shower was broken. He asked if he could come in and use mine.

'Go for it, mate,' I said, as I settled onto the edge of the bed and reached for my iPhone. About the time that I heard the shower go on, I heard Fiona say hello.

'Everyone's out,' I said. 'Everyone.'

'I know,' she told me. 'That's wonderful. I am so happy for you. And for the kids. The news is everywhere.'

I was excited. I was exhausted. I was equally spent and bubbly. I had so much adrenaline running around, I can't remember exactly what I said. But as I started talking, I hardly took a breath.

How happy I was for all the children. How great the other rescuers were. The funny story of how I thought the coach was another one of the boys. 'A couple of the players were bigger than he was,' I marvelled. 'I swear, he could have been fifteen.' I mentioned the amazing expressions of warmth and camaraderie as soon as the mission was done.

'We had a few beers,' I told Fiona. That must have been obvious to her. 'I'm all pumped up.'

As I spoke, Fiona mostly listened. She just kept saying things like 'aw' and 'wonderful' and 'that's so great'.

I know now that her mind was racing and she was looking for a place to break in. But she let me keep on talking until I had run out of puff.

Then, finally she said: 'There's something else. It's your dad.'

It was her tone of voice as much as the words she said. I grasped her message immediately. My father was dead.

Talk about a head-on collision of clashing emotions. With so much already crowding my head, I didn't know if I could process this at all.

'What happened?' I asked.

As Fiona got the story from Amanda, my father had seemed back to his normal self. He had left his room at the nursing home that evening and gone down to the dining room in his pyjamas to tell the gang he was having dinner in his room. The nurse offered him a cuppa at 7.15, then returned at 7.45 to find him on the floor.

He looked perfectly peaceful. He was dead.

I could only imagine how tough it was for Fiona, holding that news in as long as she did, so I could share my blast of exuberance and get my stories out. Waiting for just the right moment. Not wanting to step on my stories. Not wanting to spoil my excitement and relief. Giving me all the space I needed to decompress. But also knowing that she couldn't wait till morning. Knowing she had to tell me now.

It was only ten minutes or so, but it must have been the longest ten minutes of Fiona's life. She sat on the phone with me, knowing what she knew, until I was finally ready to hear it.

Just then, Craig came out of the shower.

He took one glance in my direction. I managed a quick, 'See you, mate. See you in the morning.' He didn't linger. I didn't want him to see me blubbing.

As Craig headed back to his room, I collapsed on the bed. I'd just had four of the most emotional days of my life – and now *this*? I broke down completely. Poor Fiona had to listen to me sobbing on the phone.

We all knew Dad wouldn't live forever. He was walking around on borrowed time. I knew he had been following the reports from Thailand on the TV news with steady updates when Amanda and others went to visit. They brought him the local paper, *The Advertiser*, which featured my ugly mug on the front page one of the days. I can only imagine how he was bragging to the staff and the other residents that his son was over there. I can't say my dad was ready to go.

Honestly, it would have been nice if we'd got a warning before the end. Long enough to gather around one last time, say how much we loved him and deliver our goodbyes. We had that with Mum when she got near the end.

Given his terrible family history and his pleasure-first lifestyle, he easily could have left us half a century earlier, when he was smoking and drinking and putting on weight. He'd have only been following a Harris-family tradition. I am grateful he managed to skip all that.

I told Craig the next morning at breakfast. Craig's not famous for being emotional, but I was touched by his kind words. 'Mate,' he said, 'I'm really sorry. I guess you'll need to get straight home?' Beyond that, I didn't announce anything. Really what would I have said? *Sorry to bring everyone down, but my father just died?*

When I did step outside, the triumph of the rescue was everywhere. In the media. On the footpath. In the marketplace. Everyone was smiling. It was like a load had been lifted off the entire nation, off the entire world. It made me feel nice to know that I had played a part. But my father's death wouldn't stay secret for long.

Glen McEwen, the Australian Federal Police manager for Asia, came up to me as we were standing outside the hotel. He's a big man, friendly and gregarious. I could tell he knew, and I got a bit teary. He just gave me this giant bear hug, and that was it. I really cried. Biting my lip, I thought, *What an unbelievably nice fellow.* I just needed a hug at that moment. This important, international police official recognised that I was a bit on the edge. He stepped up and did the job.

'Prime Minister Turnbull wants to have a Skype call with the Australians who were directly involved in the rescue,' Glen said. 'He especially wants to say hello to you.'

I didn't like the way that sounded.

'I'm not up to it,' I told Glen.

Glen said it was important. The embassy staffers, the federal police, the DFAT guys – they would all be there.

'I might lose it if he says something to me,' I told Glen. 'That won't look too good. Tell him not to single me out.'

Glen agreed to pass the message on.

They'd set up a laptop for the Skype call in a tiny hotel room. As the others gathered around, I hid in the back of the crowd, as inconspicuously as I could. A minute or two later, Malcolm Turnbull came on the screen from Canberra. The way he sounded, he could have been right next door.

'Good morning, everyone,' he said cheerfully, then added straightaway: 'Is Dr Harris there?'

Oh, no!

Suddenly, all these big coppers were shuffling me to the front and sitting me down, dead centre to the camera lens.

'Good morning, sir,' I said.

'I'm sorry for your loss,' the prime minister declared.

Oh, you're killing me, I was thinking. But I didn't say that. Even I could see the humour here. He'd been told not to bring it up. But the first thing out of his mouth was: 'Is Dr Harris there?' I guess he couldn't help himself.

He and I had a nice chat. It was fine. After he wished everyone well and we said our goodbyes, one of the people from DFAT came over to me. 'Look,' he said. 'This news is going to get out. Do you want us to do something? We can tell the media about your father and just ask them to be respectful. I can't promise they will, but we can ask.'

'Yeah, whatever you think is best,' I said.

It was amazing how quickly that news spread.

Julie Bishop, the foreign-affairs minister, said something, and there it was, in the little words crawling across the bottom on the CNN screen.

'Cave rescuer's father dies in Australia. Jim Harris, Adelaide surgeon.'

But I have to say it made me smile.

Dad's on the telly! It really would have tickled him. He would have loved that.

The news about my father couldn't help but cast a shadow on how I was feeling that first day and the days that followed. After the phone call with Fiona, I managed not to cry again. I just started saying to people, 'Thanks very much, but don't be too nice to me. I don't want to blub. Let's move on.'

And soon enough, I was also able to see the happy side of it. The kids were all out of the cave. My father had died the way he wanted to. I was happy for them and for him. Any pity on my part was entirely selfish now. Lots of people said what Craig had said: 'We presume you'll want to go home right away.' But I thought, 'No, I don't think that would be the right thing to do. I'm going to stay around for a few days. I need to debrief with all these guys. It's really important to spend a bit of time with the people I've shared this experience with and get to know them in a bit more normal circumstances.'

So I said, 'No, I'll stick around until Friday. I think it's good to celebrate. My father, if anyone, would understand.'

25

High Fives

Harry

'We'd really just like to walk around town and relax,' I said to the ever-vigilant Michael Costa. I was hoping that by now, even Michael would feel like he was off-duty. 'Maybe we can have a coffee and go to the market. Be normal tourists for a day.'

That seemed like a harmless request. Not to our DFAT minders, it didn't. I'm not sure what they were still so jumpy about. There were no more rescues left to botch, no home governments left to embarrass. All of Mae Sai was in a thoroughly celebratory mood. The Wild Boars' cave drama was the biggest thing that had happened around here since – well, since *ever*. And it had turned out splendidly. The town was still crawling with hundreds of foreigners, rescuers and media types, many of whom would soon be testing the limits of their company expense accounts. It was like the circus had come to town, and the elephants all had black American Express cards. Yes, northern Thailand is a serene, cultural, deeply spiritual place, but people still need to eat. Everyone, it seemed, had something to smile about. But Michael and his clipboard were still a bit concerned. He asked Kittanu to escort us on our stroll-about.

'How about a haircut?' Craig asked.

That sounded like an excellent place to start. Both of us looked a little shabby, even after a shower and a decent sleep. The exhaustion, both physical and emotional, had caught up with me, and I don't think I tossed or turned once. I figured there was some chance we'd be in the media so I didn't want to look too ratty for the folks back home. Anyway, I enjoy getting haircuts in odd places!

Kittanu led us into a small barber shop run by a beautiful old Thai lady. She gave both of us very sharp haircuts, and that wasn't even the best part. When she was done cutting, she performed fantastic head and neck massages.

'Gawd,' I moaned. 'This is so good. After four days in that bloody cave, this is unbelievable.'

Craig, not usually a great fan of a massage, reluctantly agreed. For the first time, I wasn't thinking about the dozens of ways we could have messed this up or that we really could have ended up behind bars in the Bangkok Hilton or that my whole medical practice could have been wrecked when I became known as the doctor who killed those Thai kids.

The woman at the barber shop asked for 50 baht from each of us, not much more than two dollars Australian. We each gave her a 500-baht note.

Over the next day and a half, Craig and I could finally do something we hadn't been able to do since we left Australia. We could finally relax. We needed it. We deserved it, didn't we?

With all that had been happening, we'd hardly had time to

take a breath. It's a little hard to relax when you're holding the lives of thirteen human beings in your hands and the whole world is watching, waiting to see whether you are going to succeed or fail. Until we cleared the cave and had a few hours to let the tension evaporate, I didn't fully realise just how much pressure we'd all been under. But now that our work was done, I wasn't sure which was more intense: the feeling of utter elation or the feeling of utter relief.

The celebrating began even before the sun went down. It started with a lavish poolside barbecue at Le Méridien Chiang Rai Resort, an elegant riverside hotel with lush gardens and beautiful grounds. The American PJs were there. So were the Brits and the Europeans and a bunch of other people besides. I did wonder about Lumberjack, Snuff, Fitz and the other Australian Federal Police officers we'd met along the way. Maybe they'd show up later. The hotel laid out a fantastic spread of food and copious beer and spirits. No one could stop smiling, it seemed.

Around eight o'clock, someone yelled out: 'We're all going to the general's house!' I didn't know who the general was or where he lived or what he had to do with any of this. But we all jumped into the vans that were parked outside and were driven to a big outdoor restaurant. I didn't know what happened to the general until I realised he was up on stage with the Thai country and western band, singing John Denver's 'Take Me Home, Country Roads' at the top of his voice! The restaurant had a huge buffet of spicy Thai food and beautiful Thai 'Singha girls' plying us with frosty beers. It was all a bit surreal but the perfect environment for a good old-fashioned debrief. We kept eating and kept drinking and started singing along with the general's country band. Then, someone yelled out again: 'Now we're off to the biggest disco in Thailand!'

Why stop now?

We all piled back into the vans and took another drive. Again, I had no idea where we were going. But other people seemed to, and that was good enough for us. We were also supposed to be staying at a new hotel that night. I had no idea where that was either. But I figured we'd worry about that later. The next thing I knew, Craig and I were in a massive nightclub, where a boy band was playing, lights were flashing and people were drinking and dancing wildly and carrying on. The place was packed and so loud you had to shout to be heard. The Americans, the British, the Europeans – everyone in our group seemed to be going strong, as more people kept coming over, shaking our hands and thanking us. I don't know how so many people knew who we were. Maybe they'd seen us on television? But they definitely seemed to know us.

About one in the morning, I abruptly realised we were well and truly over the edge. 'We've gotta get back to the hotel,' I said – make that *slurred* – to Craig.

Craig, who'd had as many beers and scotches as I had, nodded in a way that I interpreted as agreement.

We snaked through the crowd and more congratulations and managed to find our way outside. Only then did the thought occur to me: *Oh, right. We don't know where we're staying. We don't know how we're getting there. Does anyone know where our gear and our clothes are?*

It was really late, and we'd had a whole, whole lot to drink.

Normally, this is not a good situation to be in.

'Craig,' I said. 'Where the fuck are we?'

Clearly, Craig didn't know any more than I did.

'Thailand?' he deadpanned.

That's a start, I thought. In the condition that I was in, it passed for an astute observation, though maybe not all that helpful in our predicament.

But as soon as we hit the footpath, things started happening, as if by magic. Two men hustled over and led us into a van, and off we went into the warm Chiang Rai night. Who were these men? Where were they taking us? We did not know. But after one last drive, we pulled into a hotel we'd never seen before. It was plush and beautiful, much nicer than the border-side joint where we'd been staying, and somehow all our stuff was already in our rooms.

I really don't remember much after that. I went to bed, I suppose.

The next morning, Craig and I did make it to breakfast, though we both felt a bit quiet. Glen McEwen sauntered over to our table and said cheerfully: 'Morning, boys. How are you?'

'Not bad,' Craig said. 'No idea whatsoever how we got home last night though.'

The chief smiled at that. 'Well,' he said, 'see those blokes over there?'

He pointed towards a table where half a dozen Thai police officers were finishing breakfast. They looked far more alert than we did as they smiled and waved in our direction. We waved back.

'Do you know who they are?' the chief asked.

We shook our heads no.

'They're the Thai tourist police. They were with you all night last night. You didn't know that? They were making sure you didn't do anything you or our country might regret. They were the ones who got you home.'

That just figured.

Here we were, thinking we were a couple of crazy guys out on the town in Chiang Rai, having the time of our lives, and we actually had babysitters the whole time. Not the image we were going for.

*

The boys were all at Chiangrai Prachanukroh Hospital, where they had been taken variously by helicopter or ambulance. I'm not sure whether that included the vehicle that Craig and I had commandeered to dodge the Thai prime minister. But I was eager to see the kids in the hospital. I felt I needed to follow them up and to close the loop on my doctor–patient relationship. I asked Kittanu to try to organise a visit for Craig and me.

'When can we come in and see them?' I pressed. 'I'd really appreciate it.'

Initially, it seemed like it might not happen at all. 'Not even the parents are being allowed to go in,' Kittanu reported back. 'The boys are in some kind of quarantine.'

Quarantine?

I wasn't sure exactly what that meant under these circumstances or why it might be necessary. As far as I knew, the boys shouldn't have any communicable diseases. Everything we'd been hearing said they were doing fine. And if they needed to be isolated because of a cave-borne illness or some other exotic threat, why didn't Craig and I need to be quarantined too? We'd been roaming all over the market and the nightclubs with no restrictions placed on us. I can tell you this much: If a dozen Australian children had been trapped in a cave for seventeen days and they finally got out, there'd be a riot if their parents were told to stay away. Aussie mums and dads would be busting through the windows and kicking down the doors to hug their children. In fact, I don't believe these wrung-out Thai parents were allowed to hold their kids for three days after the last child was rescued.

But by early afternoon, we got the word. We could drop into the hospital if we wanted to.

Chiangrai Prachanukroh is large and impressive: 756 beds, founded in 1937, affiliated with the medical school at Navamindradhiraj

University. It's the premier health-care institution for Chiang Rai Province. After arriving in the DFAT van, Craig and I were greeted by a stern-looking woman in a green military uniform who was introduced to us as 'the matron'. She was polite but didn't give the appearance of someone who was used to putting up with any nonsense. She could well have been packing some concealed weapon, ready to deploy if we caused any trouble.

There were some parents upstairs. But they weren't with their children. They were staring through a window on the far side of a locked door, a set-up you might see in a neonatal intensive-care unit or maybe a facility for the criminally insane. All the parents could do was gaze in at their sons. They couldn't go in there and touch their children, whom they'd been separated from for more than two emotionally gruelling weeks.

'What's that about?' Craig grumbled as we walked the busy hallway to the boys.

I'm not sure who was making these decisions, whether it was the hospital administration or the Thai leadership. Those power centres aren't easy to tell apart. Were the powers-that-be so eager to be seen doing something, this was what they had decided to do? But it was their country. They had their own ways of doing things. Maybe they had their reasons, I don't know. We weren't looking to argue with anyone. We just wanted to check on the boys and wish them well.

The hospital staffers were welcoming to Craig and me in a formal sort of way. They seemed fine with my wearing shorts, a T-shirt and boots but insisted we both pull on surgical masks before they led us into a large open ward, where Coach Ekk and the boys were lying in hospital beds in matching, loose-fitting white-print gowns with surgical masks on their faces or dangling around their necks.

There were TVs on, and some of the boys had hand-held video-game consoles. It was lunch time, and every boy had a tray with four or five bowls of food and a plastic squirt-bottle of hand sanitiser.

The way they were shovelling that food down, they looked like they hadn't eaten a proper meal in a couple of weeks, which was actually true.

Their smiles were brilliant.

We walked from bed to bed.

'Hello.'

'G'day.'

'Hello.'

Everyone said 'hello' back to us in English and also greeted us in the traditional Thai manner, with a head-bowing *wai*. When Craig or I asked how they were feeling or what they'd had to eat in the hospital or what was the first thing they wanted to do when they got home, a woman translated for us.

We made our way around the sterile white room, stopping at each and every bed, trading small-talk and shaking the boys' little warm hands.

We spent some extra time with Adul, the one boy who spoke some English. He was eager to tell us how he and his teammates had reacted when they first realised they were trapped in the cave.

'The water blocked our way,' Adul said, holding his hands out in front of him to demonstrate. 'When we tried to leave, we couldn't go out. Then, the water kept rising, and we had to run back into the cave and find a higher place to go.'

The team members spent the first night in an area that sounded like chamber 8. 'But the water was still coming up the next morning,' Adul said. 'So we had to go more far. That was the high place where we stayed until Dr Harry jabbed us and made us sleep and sent us out.'

Having been in both those locations, I found it fascinating to hear a child's perspective. Actually, it didn't sound so different from what we had experienced, just a lot quicker.

I didn't conduct any medical examinations on the boys, but none of them appeared unhealthy at all, beyond the random sniffles and scratchy throats you'd find in any middle-school class. And if outside germs were such a pressing concern, no one said anything about my boots, which were still caked in cave mud.

It was great to see that some of the boys felt strong enough to sit up on the edge of their beds to greet us. Coach Ekk, still the leader, was all smiles and seemed extra-pleased. After a warm bow, he grinned widely and gave me a strong handshake, looking deeply into my eyes. Even with an international team of hundreds of military and civilian volunteers, it was Ekk, in those early days, who had shouldered the responsibility of caring for these children completely on his own. I believe he saved their lives before anyone else had a chance to. It was hard to hold back the tears in my emotionally fragile state.

I expected the boys to be shy around us, but they actually seemed fairly exuberant. Direct eye contact. Big, broad smiles. They all appeared to remember who we were, even though they'd only ever seen us in full diving gear. No one seemed to object to us being there before their parents. It was all a bit stilted, but it still felt amazing being with them. We'd experienced something extraordinary together, something genuinely death-defying, and all of us had come through alive. That was something we would share always.

Minutes later, I turned around and saw Pak, somehow making the same hospital gown look sharp, striding right towards me. He came to a stop just in front of me. Then, spontaneously, without saying a word, we enveloped each other in a big bear-hug. The connection

I felt with this doctor, it was almost overwhelming to me. I couldn't easily express my gratitude at having another medical man in the cave with me, someone to share the burden of this grave undertaking we had both embarked on. He was just a phenomenal bloke. We had counted on each other so much. He was the one who did most of the interpreting in the cave. He was the other, true grown-up. He was always smiling, always happy, always upbeat, the consummate role model and leader. Clear, calm, focused – a natural motivator. I could understand why his troops were so fond of him and why the boys seemed to trust him unreservedly. He exuded the sense that, as long as he was with you, everything was going to be fine.

I felt like Pak and I would be friends for the rest of our lives. Apparently, he felt the same.

When we finished visiting with Pak and the boys, a long line of nurses and doctors paraded out for us, and we got to meet all of them. We posed for photos with the medical staff and the nursing staff including the matron, who told us she was a colonel in the Royal Thai Army. That made perfect sense. But as we prepared to leave, I still felt uncomfortable. I realised I'd spent a lot of the visit worried about the lads not being permitted to reconnect with their folks. I still couldn't understand that at all.

A couple of people did mention the need to protect the boys psychologically, and I was all for that. I didn't tell anyone what I was thinking, but maybe I should have: if you really want to mess with a kid's head, put him in a cave for a couple of weeks, then don't let him see his parents after he comes out. Whatever the reasoning was – medical, political, psychological or something else – none of it made any sense to me.

As we said our final goodbyes, we also ran into the Navy SEALs who'd been with the boys in the cave. Now, they were in the corridor, about to be discharged. Maybe it was all organised, but it seemed accidental to me. I also felt a connection to them, even beyond the fact that they were Pak's guys. It wasn't so much what any of us said. None of us really said that much. But I felt like, going through what we'd all been through together, we all shared an understanding that set us apart.

Epilogue

'Healthy, Happy, Smiley'

Harry

We didn't fly commercial. Craig and I hitched a ride home on a Royal Australian Air Force transport plane, which was sent to scoop up all the Aussie government people who had helped in Thailand. They seemed perfectly happy for Craig and me to come along. Sitting in the back of this massive Boeing C-17 Globemaster III was really my first chance to reflect on the extraordinary events of the past eight days. What an adventure this had turned out to be, the diving kind and the human kind. How proud we were of all we had accomplished, even with the sad news about my dad. I know my father watched some of the rescue coverage on television. From what I heard later, everyone at the nursing home did.

Fiona and my sisters took the newspapers to him and pointed out the front-page stories. He couldn't remember all the details from one day to the next. But he seemed to grasp I was off on another of my cave-diving adventures, that this one was in Thailand and that we were trying to help some stranded children over there.

It was one of the things I had been most hoping to do as soon as I got back to Australia, drive over to the nursing home to see my dad. If I was lucky, he'd be with it enough for us to play that old why-don't-you-quit game again. I would promise I would give up the diving once and for all. He would realise I was messing with him. We would both burst out laughing.

As all of us grow older, it's rituals like those that help keep us engaged.

Nobody wanted a huge, formal funeral. Not for Jim Harris. What sense would that make? My sisters and I went to a little funeral parlour run by friends of ours. They're very nice people. They'd handled the funeral for my mother. 'We're back for another Harris,' we announced.

We had the simplest ceremony possible. About twenty of us, just close family. I said a few words and so did my sisters. Several of the grandkids stood up and spoke, my children and their cousins. They were all very close to the man they called Papa. They told funny stories about outings they'd been on with him. To them, he was always that bloke who made everyone laugh.

Then, we had the real send-off.

We rented out a room at the Feathers Hotel in Burnside. Open invitation. People telling other people, spreading by word of mouth. Hundreds – I'm not exaggerating – hundreds of people showed up, getting on the grog, telling stories and renewing old acquaintances and having unbridled fun. We started about three in the afternoon. We didn't get out of there until after 9 p.m., when I wandered over to the barman to settle up.

'Tab, please,' I said.

He poked at the screen of his register, and the full receipt began printing out and printing out and printing out. I swear that paper tape must have been four metres long.

I'd never seen a bar bill like it, but that's what I was handed that night.

'Don't worry, Dad's paying,' I said to the barman.

My dad would have loved every minute of it, every last laugh and hoisted glass. It was just a brilliant event. All his old mates were there along with the next generation and the next generation after that. Everyone was talking with everyone. No one crying, everyone laughing, people just having a grand old time. I wish Dad could have been there and Mum, too. It was a truly perfect send-off for a wonderful man.

He was eighty-eight. He had as full a life as anyone could hope for. He was a wonderful father and a treasured friend. He even got to share in his son's greatest adventure. What more could anyone ask?

All thirteen of the boys were discharged from Chiangrai Prachanukroh Hospital on Wednesday, 18 July, after a full week of quarantine, observation and many large meals. 'My own bed felt warm,' said Duangpetch Promthep, the boy known as Dom, whose first home-cooked meal was stewed pork knuckles over rice. There had been nothing like that in the cave, not even the American MREs that were so tasty that several of the boys tried to smuggle them out. Since he had turned thirteen on 3 July – one of four Wild Boars (along with Night, Nick and Note) to have a birthday in the cave – Dom finally got to blow out the candles on his belated cake.

But Thai officials were still worried about the boys. Though the coach and the players all seemed physically healthy, what about their heads? The cave experience had to have taken a mental toll, didn't it? No one could say for certain. But eleven of the boys – all except for the Christian Adul – promptly joined Coach Ekk in another kind of quarantine, a week-long Buddhist retreat at a local temple. They prayed. They meditated. Their heads were shaved. They dressed in traditional robes. They all spent time in quiet reflection. And before they returned to their families on 25 July, Coach Ekk was ordained a monk and the players novices. They dedicated their retreat to Saman Gunan, the former Thai Navy SEAL who died helping to rescue them.

Biw's mother thought all this was nice, up to a point. 'We can only do this for nine days,' she said. 'Then, he has to go back to study and prepare for exams, back to his normal life.'

Whether any of this helped to ease the boys' return to normalcy, it did achieve one thing: it kept them inaccessible to the international media. On 6 August, the boys were welcomed to Mae Sai Prasitsart School. They received new uniforms from the school management and red Bayern Munich football jerseys from a German club. Brightly coloured threads were tied around their wrists, a traditional *bai si* ritual meant to signify moral support. Then, the boys were given make-up classes for all the schoolwork they'd missed.

On 8 August, something truly momentous occurred.

A small ceremony was held in Mae Sai. Adul, Mark, Tee and Coach Ekk, the four stateless Boars, stood together at the front of the room. Each of them was promised fast-track citizenship and given a Thai national identification card. This process normally takes up to ten years, when it happens at all. This designation might not sound like much to someone who is born a citizen. But for these four and around half a million other stateless people living in Thailand, it could be life-changing. With the new ID cards, the four could travel freely, work legally in various professions and receive access to public services such as health care.

'We are very, very happy,' Tee's father, Inn Khamluang, said afterwards. The family had already been waiting for three or four years, he noted, since Tee was in the sixth grade.

The drama faded no more quickly for us.

After a day or two, I figured – a week or two max – everything that happened in Thailand would fade into the mists of history. The media would move on to the next heart-wrenching drama. People would get bored. Craig and I would have some fun stories to regale our friends with while our loved ones rolled their eyes and grumbled, 'Oh, that again.' A diving magazine might do a follow-up feature, and that would be about it. And all our lives would get back to normal – and, really, wasn't it about time?

No chance.

The reporters kept calling Craig and me and showing up at our homes. School groups and business associations invited us to speak. There was talk of books and movies and other crazy stuff. People kept using the damn H-word, and the awards started pouring in. We'd barely towelled the cave water out of our hair when important organisations started giving us awards. There was the Star of Courage, which honours 'acts of conspicuous courage in circumstances of great peril'. We were given the Medal of the Order of Australia, which is a very formal thing established in the 1970s by Queen Elizabeth II. It was a special thrill for me to receive the Edgar Pask Citation from the Association of Anaesthetists of Great Britain and Ireland, named for the medical pioneer whose bold experiments on himself in the water had so pumped up my own confidence. That was cool. But just as all the excitement seemed finally to be fading, Craig and I were named regional winners for Australian of the Year,

Craig for Western Australia, me for South Australia. The Australian of the Year is a wonderful honour that celebrates Australians who work to improve the country and the world in fields that range from science to community welfare to medicine, the environment and the arts – anything, really, that improves Australia or the planet.

In January, all thirty-two of the state winners, four from each state or territory, were invited with our families to a three-day shindig at the capital in Canberra. Well, bugger me if we didn't win. Prime Minister Scott Morrison made the announcement, keeping the suspense until the last second. Danielle Roche, who chaired the National Australia Day Council, praised our 'selflessness, courage and willingness to help others in a time of need'. She said we 'embody the very best of the Australian spirit . . . They are the people that make us proud to be Australian.'

I glanced at a stony-faced Craig as she was saying all that. He looked just as stunned as I felt. I'm not saying it wasn't nice hearing all those wonderful things about ourselves, but I am saying I kept assuming there must be some mistake. I also wanted to use the chance to raise a larger issue Craig and I had both been thinking about.

'I am proud to call myself an explorer,' I said in my acceptance speech. 'But I do fear for kids today who, living in a risk-averse society, will not learn to challenge themselves and to earn the grazed knees and stubbed toes that really are necessary to build resilience and confidence. I think a need for adventure resides in all of us. The answer for some is found in reading books and for others by watching the screen. But for others like ourselves, exploration is really an addiction. For me – or for us – it is about caves. Caves are the last place on this earth where an explorer can be the very first person to find something unique and witness something for the first time and call it our own. It is thrilling to be part of a wave of citizen scientists in that community who are revealing some of the world's secrets.

'So we must encourage children to be part of that wave of enthusiastic amateurs like ourselves. Not necessarily in caves, perhaps.'

Laughter.

'And you might think it strange, having just rescued some kids, that I would like to promote kids to come underground.'

More laughter.

'But actually kids do need to be kids, and they need to be allowed to be so. They need to be allowed to find their own boundaries and to test their own limits. So I plan to spend this year encouraging kids to do just that and to find their inner explorer. Equally importantly to ask parents to relax a little and let them have a little rope to do that.'

Applause.

'Outdoor activities really do promote physical and mental well-being. And it is critical that kids can test their own limits,' I said.

When I got finished, Craig leaned into the microphone. 'I really am somewhat astounded that the pursuit of a hobby for the last twenty-two years has led to so much interest and acknowledgement and me being up here tonight,' he began.

Craig wanted to focus on Australia. It wasn't only that this was the country honouring us. It was also that Australia was the force that had made us who we were. 'I have had the most extraordinary good fortune throughout my life,' he said. 'Probably the single greatest factor is having been born in Australia.'

I don't think anyone could argue with that.

But Craig's mind, like mine, was on the lessons here for regular people around the world, how all of us can be prepared for the next challenges to confront us. 'At an individual level,' he said, 'we must all accept personal responsibility for our destiny. Confronting the small challenges that appear every day and taking responsibility for your actions and their consequences is the only way to be ready for the life-defining events.'

Too many people hide from this, he said.

'There is a temptation to take the easy road, to think that life would be better if we mould it to be as comfortable as possible,' Craig continued. 'But there is a real and serious risk in doing this, the risk that we miss the opportunities that present themselves. Missing a chance to lend a hand and help others. A risk of never knowing our own strength and what we are capable of. And we risk that, when we face our test and adversity confronts us, we crumble into a heap and give up instead of standing up.'

Get out there and do it, we both agreed.

So what about the kids?

As far as we were concerned, that was the last, lingering question from our time in Thailand, the final piece of unfinished business we still had to attend to. From the day we left the country, Craig and I wanted to – needed to – go back and check on the boys.

How were they doing? What were they up to? Were they suffering nightmares from their time in the cave? It's an awesome responsibility when you think about it. If you help to save someone's life, you feel a strange investment in how they go on to use it. It's hard to explain exactly, but both Craig and I felt a lasting connection to these boys.

In mid-April, nine months after everyone was safely out of the cave, Craig and I were invited back to Thailand as honoured guests of the government. Fiona and Heather came along, as did Millie and Charlie. Our families had earned a nice holiday after all we'd put them through. It's no exaggeration to say we were treated like royalty every step of the way. We had lunch with Don Pramudwinai, the Thai foreign minister. Prime Minister Prayut Chan-o-cha received us along with some of the AFP and Australian Defence Force personnel. It was nice to finally shake the prime minister's hand, having snuck out on him the first time around. We must have visited a half a dozen temples. We had lights-and-sirens police escorts and one especially harrowing 162-kilometre-per-hour ride down a highway in a Toyota HiAce van, a possible land speed record for this vehicle! Even our tuk-tuk ride had a police escort.

At a highly formal ceremony in Bangkok, Craig and I were presented with the Knight Grand Cross (First Class) of the Most Admirable Order of the Direkgunabhorn, a red-gold-and-silver medal depicting a mythological Garuda bird. The medal was attached to a beautiful green sash with red, white and yellow trim. 'It is worn from the right shoulder to the left hip,' a helpful royal aide leaned over and whispered to us.

That was nice to know, but we had a lot more fun at our next stop – hanging out with Pak and drinking Singha beers in the bar of the SO/Sofitel Bangkok hotel. 'We're a long way from Tham Luang cave,' Craig commented as we gazed out the floor-to-ceiling windows across Sathorn Road towards Lumpini Park.

That first time we'd met in the cave, Pak said we'd have to meet up again one day to drink Thai beer. Well, here we were. I couldn't think of anywhere in the world I'd rather be.

In the nine months since we'd seen each other, our lives and Pak's life had picked up some unexpected similarities. Like us, he was now famous in his own country. He had been travelling constantly, giving talks and interviews. People were eager to hear from him about what had happened in the cave. 'I try to explain as well as I can,' he said.

'So do we,' Craig said.

'It's an honour and a big responsibility,' Pak continued. 'But sometimes I also wish my life could just go back to normal. Just be a father and a husband and a doctor and an Army officer.'

That lit a flash of recognition in both of us.

Pak really had turned out to be everything he seemed. Warm. Cheerful. Utterly competent and fully in charge. The military doctor from central casting. And he was still just as concerned about the wellbeing of the boys as he was when we first swam up to their muddy encampment in the cave.

'That part is gratifying,' he said. 'From everything I have heard, they seem to be doing very well. I told you they were good boys.'

Pak said his own son was also doing well. 'He missed me when I was away,' Pak said. 'But when I got home, I gave him a giant hug. I just kept looking at him. After being with the boys in the cave for so long and always thinking about my son, I couldn't stand the thought that something bad might happen to him.'

I was certain – I know Craig was too – that we would be friends with Pak forever. Across a lifetime, you don't meet many people like him. But we were still eager to head up to the scene of our great adventure and to reconnect with the boys who had found themselves caught in the middle of it all. They really were the reason we had come back to Thailand, far more than the honours and the thankyous, nice as they were. We made the short flight up to Chiang Rai and the hour-long van ride further north into Mae Sai.

Things were so much quieter now.

All the rescuers and most of the media were off in the wind somewhere. Though the interior of the cave was still closed to the public, the Tham Luang cave site had become a tourist attraction. There were maps and brochures and photos depicting the rescue. Guides were available to tell visitors the story. People were selling things. American expat Josh Morris, who had helped us navigate the Thai generals, and the prescient expat-British caver Vern Unsworth came along with us on this special return visit.

Before stepping inside, we stopped to pay our respects at a recently erected statue of Saman Gunan, the ex-Navy SEAL who died in the cave, and at a statue of the Sleeping Lady Nang Non, for whom the mountain range is named. Only then did we feel ready to revisit this place that had meant so much to all of us.

'We are not planning on being in there for any great time,' I quipped in a pre-caving media interview. 'But that's what the kids said, right?'

That got a nervous laugh. So did my plea before we all went in.

'If we are not out in four hours,' I said with a smile, 'we want you to all come in and help. Bring some chocolate and some beer.'

The cave looked very different without water in it. Some parts were easy to recognise, but other bits, which we knew only by feel, were utterly unfamiliar to us. In April, we could walk to places that only divers would be able to reach in June or July. We hiked and crawled as far as chamber 9, where Coach Ekk and the boys had spent all those days. Then, we walked a few hundred metres past there. That must have been where the assistant coach and his team had attempted to find another way out by going even deeper. They left clues. Scratched into the limestone wall with a chunk of rock were two numerals and a letter – 13p, a message that presumably indicated how many people were trapped in the cave. At a nearby spot, someone marked the date – 24 June 2018.

Craig and I would have loved to keep going, but on this visit, we had family and inexperienced cavers along. We weren't taking any chances, and we didn't have our gear. No one had to rescue any of us, not even my kids or the slightly nervous Aussie embassy staff who joined us. But even more than seeing the cave, we wanted to see Coach Ekk and the boys. We had all been impressed and inspired by them. But they weren't just symbols or media figures or Wild Boars, not to us they weren't. They were young people with hopes and dreams, challenges and opportunities and day-to-day lives. We felt an obligation to follow up with them. As divers. And as fellow human beings. We wanted to make sure they were doing okay.

I also had some questions for them, and so did Craig. In part it was out of concern and curiosity, in part to set the record straight. We wanted to know what they remembered from the rescue, what they thought of us, how they felt about our anaesthesia-diving exit plan and how they were reacting emotionally now that it was all over. We still didn't know the answers to any of that. Once and for all, we also wanted to clear up some myths that had crept into the public telling of the story of the boys in Tham Luang cave. Did they really drink water dripping from the limestone? Did they really go to the toilet in the cave water? Were they really unable to swim? The news stories had asserted all of that, over and over again. We had our doubts and wondered if the boys could set the record straight. Not sharing the same language, we had never been able to do that fully before.

We met Coach Ekk and seven of the boys at the temple. We were touched that so many of them came. We did a quick interview with the Thai media then went into another part of the temple for some private time. The coach and the boys seemed thrilled to welcome us back.

As Craig and I sat cross-legged on the floor, each of the boys came over and knelt in front of us. Hands together, they bowed. Then, in a gesture I hadn't seen before, each of them rested his head for a moment on our knees. We weren't sure how to respond to that. But quickly, the boys got up and gave us each a hug. After that, they were rambunctious young people again.

'What do you remember from the day you left the cave?' I asked them.

They all started laughing.

'Good boy, good boy! Jab, jab!'

They were mimicking the soothing blather of my pre-anaesthesia technique. They thought it was hilarious.

'Good boy, good boy! Jab, jab!'

They all remembered taking the anti-anxiety tablet and receiving the jabs. They remembered waking up in the field hospital or on the way to the big hospital in Chiang Rai. They remembered nothing in between.

'Ketamine did its job,' Craig said to me.

When I brought up the misconceptions from the media coverage, the answers came, unequivocally, in a near-chorus of boys. The story of drinking water that dripped off the rocks? Rubbish, they said. They drank cave water flowing past the bottom of the hill. It stayed clear until the divers came and stirred up the silt.

The story of the boys using the cave water like a toilet? Simply wrong. They dug holes in the dirt across the sump, swimming over with the ever-attentive Navy SEALs each time they had to go.

The assertion that the boys were unable to swim? Nonsense, they said. They went swimming often at school. Almost all of them could swim, though we had correctly believed that none of them had underwater diving experience.

'At some point,' Craig said to me, 'you really have to question everything in the story, even the things you think you saw with your own eyes. Memory is an unreliable thing.'

I had so much more I wanted to ask about, and now was the chance to ask it.

'Our plan to make you go to sleep and dive you out of the cave while you were sleeping – did that sound sensible? Or did it sound like madness?'

'It was good,' they said.

'Did you think it was dangerous?' Craig asked.

'No, we trusted you.'

That made me shudder. *We* didn't even trust us. They had no idea how perilous this was.

If somebody tells you something, you are inclined to believe it unless you have some reason not to. They had no power in the situation. It was completely beyond their control. When you are in a spot like that, you do as you are told. Trapped in the dark, deep, flooded cave with no obvious way out, what choice did these boys have?

As Craig and I had travelled around in the months since we'd left Thailand, we were constantly asked how the experience in the cave had affected the boys psychologically. We had a stock answer. We said we weren't trained to offer a serious professional judgement. But as far as we could tell from a distance, the kids seemed to be doing fine.

We were also asked if the experience had upset us. 'Why would I be upset?' I asked. 'I was doing two things I love. Cave diving and medicine. We'd been training for this, hoping something like it might happen one day. Not wishing harm on anyone, of course, but eager to use these skills to save lives if need be. This was off the scale of what we could've ever imagined. But at the end of the day, the outcome was better than we could possibly have hoped for. It was a bloody great ending.'

As Craig liked to remind me: 'And neither one of us has paid for a beer in a very long time.'

Sometimes, people seemed a bit disappointed to hear that we weren't more distressed, us and the boys. Now that we had a chance to visit with the lads in person, they seemed exactly as they had from far away, like they were happy and were enjoying themselves and were adjusting fairly well to what life had handed them. Whatever distress they were suffering, they weren't showing it.

I had theories about this. These were country kids. They grew up in a tough environment. Several of them knew what it meant to be stateless. No one had to give them a lecture on seeking adventure. When you grow up doing hard things, you are ready for the challenges of life when they come.

That was all conjecture, I know. But it was also a lesson people everywhere could stand to learn.

Acknowledgements

Craig and Harry

Book writing, like cave diving, is at heart a team sport. Before you dip so much as a toe into the literary waters, please, bring some trusted mates along. Thankfully, we had a world-class team on this latest adventure of ours, talented and generous people who helped us get our story out in the best possible manner and made the trip far more thrilling than it otherwise would have been. We are deeply grateful to all of them.

First and always, to our immediate families: Heather, Bruce, Patricia, Ray, Jenny and Bethany. Fiona, James, Charlie, Millie, Amanda and Kristina. Yes, we know how challenging life can be when you care about someone who is drawn to the insides of distant caves. But your love, support and forbearance have given us so very much to come home to.

Now that Craig calls himself retired, fresh adventure is a full-time pursuit, for which he is profoundly grateful. Harry still toils at his day (and night) jobs – but what rewarding jobs they are, caring for patients and saving lives at Specialist Anaesthetic Services, the

South Australian Ambulance Service and MedSTAR. He is especially grateful for the wise counsel of Drs James Doube and Andrew Pearce and for the patience of his long-suffering surgical colleagues, all of whom are close friends.

Thanks to our brothers and sisters in the cave-diving community, who have inspired us so often and taught us so much about this passion we share. The Cave Diving Association of Australia, the Cave Diving Group of Great Britain and Northern Ireland, the British Cave Rescue Council and the least formal, most ridiculous but highest-spirited cave-diving group on (or below) earth, the legendary Wet Mules. If you have to ask why we cave dive, you probably wouldn't understand the answer. Cave divers are some of the world's purest adventurers. We are honoured to dive in your midst.

Just reaching Thailand was an adventure in itself, and getting settled there wasn't any less so. Luckily, we had a cast of dedicated public servants easing the way for our unique, two-man AUSMAT team. These were the heroes of the Australian Department of Foreign Affairs and Trade, the Australian Federal Police, the Australian Defence Force, the National Critical Care and Trauma Response Centre, the Australian Embassy staff in Thailand and the Thai Tourist Police, our local liaison and invisible protectors. Without all the people mentioned here, those boys might never have been rescued from that cave.

By the time we arrived at Tham Luang, Vern Unsworth, Ben Reymenants, Rob Harper, John Volanthen and Rick Stanton were already on the ground. The trail these men blazed cannot be underestimated. Rick and John not only found the children and their coach alive but eloquently conveyed the gravity of the situation to the rest of the world with the help of Josh Morris. Meanwhile on the ground, the Thai and international communities showed what crisis support is all about: volunteers pouring in from everywhere to provide meteorology, geological engineering, catering, communications, media, muscle and tonnes and tonnes of equipment to lower the water and sustain the diving operations. Local climbing and rope-access workers rigged the dry cave section and scoured the bush for alternate entrances. Drilling teams pounded through nearly a kilometre of solid rock. Three brave Thai Navy Seals, plus the pitch-perfect leadership of our new friend for life, Thai Army medic Dr Bhak Loharnshoon, cared for the vulnerable Wild Boars, knowing the adults were in as much danger as the children were. When the sedated kids were ready to be dived out, that perilous journey was led by the four British aces (Rick and John with the addition of Jason Mallinson and Chris Jewell) with special support from three talented young UK divers (Connor, Josh and Jim) and four "Euro divers" (Erik, Ivan, Claus and Nikko). Working under constant, grinding pressure, these supermen never flinched once. When the players and their young coach were delivered to chamber 3, the US pararescue teams, AFP SRG divers, Aussie CD, Chinese divers and Thai Navy and Military medics assessed the kids, then whisked them out of the cave to a field hospital before moving them to the massive hospital in Chiang Rai, where the medical and nursing staffs could ensure their full recovery.

Special personal thanks to Kittanu, Michael, Cameron, Andrew, Jo and Grace of DFAT and the AFP; John Dalla-Zuanna, Peter Wolf and the other directors of the Cave Divers Association of Australia, and Glen McEwen of the AFP. Our heartfelt condolences to the family of the man who was tragically lost along the way, former Thai Navy Seal Saman Gunan.

We are fortunate to have such a powerful editorial team in our corner: Co-author Ellis Henican, whose good humour and natural-born storytelling skills have made these events as heart-pounding to read about as they were to live through. Our tireless researcher Roberta Teer, who now officially knows more about us than we know about ourselves. Transcriber Janis Spidle, who carried our raw stories one key step closer to literature. And the first-rate publishing team at Penguin Random House Australia, publishers Cate Blake and Nikki Christer, publicist Karen Reid and editor Elena Gomez, as well as copyeditor Elizabeth Cowell, who helped turn all this into a book everyone can be proud of. With attention suddenly swirling around us, Juliette Allen guided us cheerfully and strategically across an unfamiliar media landscape.

Finally thanks to our intrepid foreword writer James Cameron, who knows a thing or two about telling great stories and has been so generous in his support of ours.

One last word about Coach Ekk and the boys: Their bravery, their calm and their grace under duress has never ceased to amaze us. Their instant trust of us – a couple of scruffy, middle-aged foreigners who swam up to them one day – is a testament to their openness and decency. It may have saved all our lives. These young people are a credit to their families, their communities and the kingdom of Thailand.

We wanted to write this book to get the story straight and give credit to all those who were in some way involved in this dramatic rescue. While for some reason we have become its public face, the role we played was no more or less important than the roles played by many hundreds (perhaps thousands) of others. We consider ourselves fortunate to have possessed some skills that could be contributed to this wonderful outcome. We are endlessly honoured to be in the company of such human greatness.